Military Sexual Trauma: Current Knowledge and Future Directions

Military Sexual Trauma: Current Knowledge and Future Directions showcases the work of several prominent military sexual trauma (MST) researchers, scholars, and clinicians from across the United States. A review of existing research and original empirical findings converge to indicate that MST contributes to a range of physical health problems, complex posttraumatic responses, and other mental health consequences above and beyond the effects of other types of traumatic experiences. This collection also presents evidence suggesting that MST is often difficult to identify both within the individual military member and within the military population as a whole. Recommendations are offered for addressing this problem. In addition to the research review and empirical findings, an evolutionary framework for understanding sexual assault of women in the military is presented. Taken together, this collection of works may inform MST intervention and prevention efforts.

This book was originally published as a special issue of *Journal of Trauma & Dissociation.*

Carolyn B. Allard, PhD, is Assistant Professor in the Department of Psychiatry at UC San Diego and Program Director of the Military Sexual Trauma Clinic at the VA San Diego Healthcare System. Her research interests include modulators of the relationship between prior trauma and posttraumatic distress following later trauma, revictimization, and treatment outcomes.

Melissa Platt, MA, MS is a doctoral candidate in clinical psychology at the University of Oregon. She is a member of Jennifer J. Freyd's Dynamics Lab focusing on interpersonal trauma. She is particularly interested in posttraumatic shame and its consequences and treatment. Melissa obtained her MA in counselling psychology from Boston College.

Military Sexual Trauma: Current Knowledge and Future Directions

Edited by

Carolyn B. Allard and Melissa Platt

Routledge
Taylor & Francis Group
LONDON AND NEW YORK

First published 2012
by Routledge
4 Park Square, Milton Park, Abingdon, Oxon, OX14 4RN

Simultaneously published in the USA and Canada
by Routledge
605 Third Avenue, New York, NY 10017

Routledge is an imprint of the Taylor & Francis Group, an informa business

This book is a reproduction of the *Journal of Trauma & Dissociation*, vol. 12, issue 3. The Publisher requests to those authors who may be citing this book to state, also, the bibliographical details of the special issue on which the book was based.

British Library Cataloguing in Publication Data
A catalogue record for this book is available from the British Library

ISBN13: 978-0-415-69681-4 (hbk)

Typeset in Times New Roman
by Taylor & Francis Books

Publisher's Note
The publisher would like to make readers aware that the chapters in this book may be referred to as articles as they are identical to the articles published in the special issue. The publisher accepts responsibility for any inconsistencies that may have arisen in the course of preparing this volume for print.

Contents

INTRODUCTION

MELISSA PLATT, MA, MS
Department of Psychology, University of Oregon, Eugene, Oregon, USA

CAROLYN B. ALLARD, PhD
Psychology Service, Department of Veterans Affairs Medical Center, and Department of Psychiatry, University of California, San Diego, California, USA

Until recently, the study of psychological effects of military trauma has focused nearly exclusively on the consequences of combat-related stressors such as being in the line of fire, experiencing an explosion, or suffering a physical injury. Meanwhile, sexual trauma has primarily been recognized in the forms of childhood or adult civilian abuse. Combat-related distress has largely been investigated among men, whereas sexual assault research has focused on women. As military sexual trauma (MST) bridges the gap between traumatic events historically divided between military and civilian and also between events traditionally categorized as happening to men versus women, its recognition may potentially represent a turning point in the field of traumatic stress.

One of the aims we had in putting together this special issue was to provide MST researchers and clinicians with a summary of the state of MST research and a collection of some of the most up-to-date MST-related investigations representative of the directions in which this research is heading. This collection is by no means exhaustive. Many other important submissions could not be included in this special issue because of space limitations. Another aim was to facilitate continued research efforts by elucidating the gaps in the extant MST research, presenting important lines of research that have begun, and proposing new areas of research that may have important implications for efforts toward preventing MST and reducing its aftermath.

The first set of papers in this special issue suggest a need for increased standardization in the study of MST prevalence and greater attention to individual differences, population selection, and measurement issues. As Allard, Nunnink, Gregory, Klest, and Platt (this issue) report, although most of what is known about MST relates to prevalence and health correlates, a high degree of unreliability in prevalence data persists. As noted by Murdoch and colleagues (this issue), the military's "gold standard" assessment of MST was normed on college-educated women and thus does not reliably capture MST rates in men or individuals without at least a college education. Hoyt, Rielage, and Williams (this issue) remind the reader that the majority of MST incidents involving male victims are not reported. Valdez and colleagues (this issue) present findings indicating that victims of MST may be overrepresented not only in posttraumatic stress disorder treatment settings but also in psychosocial rehabilitation centers and substance use treatment settings.

Despite the difficulties in assessing the absolute prevalence of MST, it is clear that it is experienced by a substantial number of women and men, with devastating outcomes. Empirical work presented in this issue demonstrates that MST is linked not only with symptoms of posttraumatic stress disorder but also with more complex posttraumatic reactions, including difficulties with interpersonal relationships, emotion regulation, dissociation, somatization, and self-perception (Luterek, Bittinger, & Simpson, this issue), increased pain-related physical health problems (Smith et al., this issue), and higher rates of trading sex (Strauss et al., this issue). What is more, these latest findings add to existing evidence, summarized in this issue by Allard and colleagues, that MST is associated with greater posttraumatic difficulties compared to other potentially traumatic experiences, including combat experiences and adult and civilian sexual abuse. Like combat trauma, MST often strips victims of their sense of safety and competence. However, unlike the MST victim, the victim of combat trauma may rely on the support of unit members and a sense of shared experience in order to cope. As noted by many of the authors in this special issue, MST is frequently accompanied by expectations of silence. Empirical study of the effects of institutional silencing and other factors purported to put MST survivors at increased risk for posttraumatic distress relative to other types of trauma is called for.

MST prevention research is equally sparse, as Allard and colleagues' (this issue) review reveals. Potentially informative to prevention efforts is Hannagan and Arrow's (this issue) evolutionary framework for understanding the sexual assault of women in the military, which is based on their review of theory and research in evolutionary principles, group and war psychology, and MST case studies. Their framework provides a guide for future research and cultural-level interventions aimed at the prevention of

MST. Empirical evidence of treatment effectiveness for MST-related distress is also limited (see Allard et al., this issue). As MST involves the unique stressors associated with a war zone environment *and* those associated with interpersonal betrayal, existing intervention efforts based on other types of traumatic experiences must be systematically empirically evaluated prior to their implementation with MST survivors.

We hope this special issue provides an impetus for increased research aimed at assessing the effectiveness of current treatments in MST populations, development of treatments that can address the myriad difficulties associated with MST, and increasing access to effective treatments for individuals experiencing distress related to MST. Some authors in the current issue offer recommendations for increasing access. Valdez and colleagues recommend resource allocation to settings where MST is overreported, including settings with high rates of MST among men. Hoyt et al. recommend MST screenings in medical settings in order to provide a safe space for disclosure among male veterans who may be avoiding mental health treatment settings.

Taken together, the findings presented in this special issue suggest that more work is needed in order to increase the reliability of MST prevalence estimates; illuminate the reasons why MST's adverse impact exceeds that of other types of traumatic experiences; better understand the male experience of MST; and inform and test prevention and intervention efforts at the individual, group, and institutional levels. Recent advances in MST awareness, including universal Veterans Health Administration screening, have made possible much of the research conducted on MST, including the publication of the important articles in this special issue. It is our hope that ongoing Veterans Health Administration support and the kinds of research efforts showcased in this collection will provide momentum for additional progress through systematic investigations of MST prevalence, prevention, and treatment outcomes to continue to inform and advance the field of traumatic stress.

Unreliability and Error in the Military's "Gold Standard" Measure of Sexual Harassment by Education and Gender

MAUREEN MURDOCH, MD, MPH
Center for Chronic Disease Outcome Research, Department of Medicine, Minneapolis VA Medical Center, and Department of Internal Medicine, University of Minnesota Medical School, Minneapolis, Minnesota, USA

JOHN B. PRYOR, PhD
Department of Psychology, Illinois State University–Normal, Normal, Illinois, USA

JOAN M. GRIFFIN, PhD
Center for Chronic Disease Outcome Research, Department of Medicine, Minneapolis VA Medical Center, and Department of Internal Medicine, University of Minnesota Medical School, Minneapolis, Minnesota, USA

DIANE COWPER RIPLEY, PhD
HSR&D/RR&D Rehabilitation Outcomes Research Center, North Florida/South Georgia Veterans Health System, Gainesville, Florida, USA

GARY D. GACKSTETTER, PhD, MPH, DVM
Analytic Services, Inc. (ANSER), Arlington, Virginia; and Uniformed Services University of the Health Sciences, Bethesda, Maryland, USA

Funding for this study was provided by the Department of Veterans Affairs (VA) Health Services Research and Development (HSR&D) Service (IIR 96-014). Drs. Murdoch, Griffin, and Polusny are core investigators for the Center for Chronic Disease Outcomes Research (CCDOR). CCDOR is a VA HSR&D Service Center of Excellence. The authors thank two anonymous reviewers for their helpful critiques. The views, opinions, and findings are the authors' and do not necessarily reflect the views of the Departments of Veterans Affairs or Defense.

MELISSA A. POLUSNY, PhD
Center for Chronic Disease Outcome Research, Departments of Psychology and Psychiatry, Minneapolis VA Medical Center, and Department of Psychiatry, University of Minnesota Medical School, Minneapolis, Minnesota, USA

JAMES S. HODGES, PhD
Division of Biostatistics, University of Minnesota, Minneapolis, Minnesota, USA

The Department of Defense's "gold standard" sexual harassment measure, the Sexual Harassment Core Measure (SHCore), is based on an earlier measure that was developed primarily in college women. Furthermore, the SHCore requires a reading grade level of 9.1. This may be higher than some troops' reading abilities and could generate unreliable estimates of their sexual harassment experiences. Results from 108 male and 96 female soldiers showed that the SHCore's temporal stability and alternate-forms reliability was significantly worse (a) in soldiers without college experience compared to soldiers with college experience and (b) in men compared to women. For men without college experience, almost 80% of the temporal variance in SHCore scores was attributable to error. A plain language version of the SHCore had mixed effects on temporal stability depending on education and gender. The SHCore may be particularly ill suited for evaluating population trends of sexual harassment in military men without college experience.

Sexual harassment, reported by up to 74% to 80% of active duty men and women (Bastian, Lancaster, & Reyst, 1996; Rosen & Martin, 1998), has been associated with symptoms of depression, anxiety, and posttraumatic stress disorder (e.g., Kang, Dalager, Mahan, & Ishii, 2005); diminished job satisfaction and performance; and even poorer nonwork interpersonal relationships (Pryor, 1995). Progress in reducing military sexual harassment has primarily been gauged by periodically surveying troops and comparing their reports of sexual harassment to those of previously surveyed troops. However, earlier sexual harassment surveys yielded widely differing prevalence estimates across service branches, primarily because each branch defined and measured sexual harassment differently. Consequently, in 1998 the Deputy Assistant Secretary of Defense for Equal Opportunity mandated the development of a standardized sexual harassment instrument that was to be "used in all [Department of Defense] and Service-wide surveys" (Lipari & Lancaster,

2003, p. 97). The military's chosen measure, the Sexual Harassment Core Measure (SHCore; Stark, Chernyshenko, Lancaster, Drasgow, & Fitzgerald, 2002), is a 12-item derivative of the Sexual Experiences Questionnaire (SEQ; Fitzgerald et al., 1988).

The SEQ was developed primarily in college students and faculty (Fitzgerald et al., 1988; Gelfand, Fitzgerald, & Drasgow, 1995), and most of its psychometric evaluation has been conducted in women (Fitzgerald, Gelfand, & Drasgow, 1995; Gelfand et al., 1995). In the armed forces, however, men outnumber women by a ratio of 6:1. Yet most psychometric evaluation of the Department of Defense's SEQ version has either excluded men or, when men were included, evaluated only a subset of the SEQ items they responded to (Fitzgerald, Magley, Drasgow, & Waldo, 1999). The SEQ/SHCore's performance in military men therefore remains uncertain.

Furthermore, perhaps because the SEQ was developed in college populations, it and the SHCore require relatively high reading grade levels of 9.8 and 9.1, respectively, based on the Flesch-Kincaide readability formula (Kincaid, Fishburne, Rogers, & Chisson, 1975). Because military recruits have on average an 11th-grade reading proficiency—which is higher than that of the general U.S. population—most military members would likely find the SHCore reasonably straightforward and easy to read. However, a substantial fraction with below-average reading skills might struggle to comprehend it. For example, approximately 10% of military troops have not completed high school, and about a third have cognitive aptitude scores between the 30th and 50th percentiles of national norms (Department of Defense, 2004). Consequently, many military training materials are targeted to a 5th- or 6th-grade reading level, which is the level literacy experts recommend to ensure comprehension of printed materials (Doak, Doak, & Root, 1996).

As with training materials, survey instruments need to perform adequately at all levels of reading comprehension. Otherwise, common results include low survey returns and more satisficed responses. Low response rates have been previously reported in military studies using the SHCore (Bastian et al., 1996), but no study has evaluated possible satisficing. "Satisficed" responses are the opposite of "optimized" responses and occur when survey respondents do not carefully and accurately interpret questions, do not fully develop an accurate summary judgment in response to questions, or do not transcribe their judgments correctly (Krosnick, 1991). They are responses that, on the face of it, appear valid but do not actually convey accurate information. Examples of extreme satisficing include endorsing the same response to every item regardless of the item content or randomly endorsing various responses for different items.

Satisficing has also been linked to poor motivation (Krosnick et al., 2002; Lam & Bengo, 2003). Military men, who generally face lower risks for sexual harassment than military women (Bastian et al., 1996; Culbertson, Rosenfeld, & Newell, 1993; Lipari & Lancaster, 2003), could be less motivated than women to respond accurately to sexual harassment questions. Furthermore, some critics have questioned the applicability and saliency of the various versions of the SEQ to men, arguing that several types of experiences important to them, such as challenges to one's masculinity, are not captured (Berdahl, Magley, & Waldo, 1996; Waldo, Berdahl, & Fitzgerald, 1998).

Whether arising from comprehension problems or low motivation, satisficed responses may increase both random and systematic measurement error (Krosnick, 1991; Krosnick et al., 2002). This in turn could cause investigators to over- or underestimate the prevalence of military sexual harassment in selected subgroups and could hinder the appropriate allocation of resources to those subgroups (e.g., to prevent the occurrence of sexual harassment or its sequelae). In addition to possible differences in sexual harassment reporting by gender, for example, satisficing could plausibly account for some of the inverse association described between years of formal education and reporting sexual harassment (Antecol & Cobb-Clark, 2006). Clarifying the SHCore's performance in groups at higher risk for satisficing is therefore important.

Because the SHCore was derived from a scale developed primarily in female college populations, we hypothesized that soldiers without college experience would be more likely to satisfice on the SHCore compared to soldiers with college experience, and military men would be more likely to satisfice compared to military women. We also hypothesized that a plain language version of the SHCore, written at a lower reading grade level, would diminish satisficing. Simpler text tends to improve reading comprehension across all reading abilities, even among those with very high reading proficiency (Doak et al., 1996), and it can sometimes counter low motivation problems by reducing cognitive burden (Krosnick, 1991).

As is common in this field, we tested these hypotheses by examining various aspects of test reliability (Krosnick et al., 2002). Test reliability is the fraction of total variance in test scores accounted for by true subject differences divided by the total test score variance, where total test score variance is the sum of variance from true subject differences and error (Guyatt, Walter, & Norman, 1987). Because satisficing increases error (i.e., increases the denominator), reliability is diminished (Krosnick et al., 2002). Thus, if satisficing related to reading comprehension is present, then soldiers without college experience should have lower internal consistency, temporal stability, alternate-forms reliability, and case concordance (kappa) on the SHCore compared to soldiers with college experience. If men are less motivated than women to optimize their responses to sexual harassment questions, these same parameters should likewise be lower in men than in women. By extension, any differences between those with and without college experience and between men and women should be reduced when a more simply written SHCore version is used. As a further check of our hypotheses, we used a measure of problem drinking written at a fourth-grade reading level to see whether satisficing and unreliable self-report were specific to the SHCore or were a more general characteristic of our sample. If satisficing were specific to the SHCore, then we expected the drinking measure's internal consistency and test–retest reliability to not differ by education or gender.

METHODS

Setting and Sample

The Minneapolis VA Medical Center's Human Studies Subcommittee reviewed and approved the study protocol, as did the relevant Army installation's commanding officer and division equal opportunity office. The study's primary goal was to examine the psychometric performance of the Department of Defense's sexual harassment measure, its plain language revision, and several other measures not discussed here.

In October 1999, a convenience sample of 108 active duty enlisted men and 96 active duty enlisted women at the same installation and for the most part in their first duty tour (mean service length = 3.1 years, *SD* = 2.7) completed a consent document and a 21-page questionnaire on site (Time 1). On the basis of their availability 1 month later, 86 participants (42% of the original sample) were invited to complete the questionnaire a second time (Time 2). On both occasions participants were offered food while completing the survey as well as a $10 gift certificate. The refusal rate for each test administration was less than 1%.

Measures

Sexual harassment. Participants completed the Department of Defense's original 26-item SEQ version (Fitzgerald et al., 1999) from which the SHCore was derived and a 31-item plain language version we created by unbundling several double- and triple-barreled items and by simplifying each item's language. We counterbalanced the order of appearance of two SEQ versions in the questionnaire. Both SEQ versions were prefielded to focus groups of active duty troops at the same Army post. Whereas officers in the focus groups tended to prefer the original version because it more clearly described unwelcome behaviors, junior enlisted soldiers tended to favor the plain language version because it was more understandable. Junior enlisted personnel found the original SEQ's preamble confusing and wordy, and they appeared to have difficulty meaningfully distinguishing among the five original response categories, which were "never," "once or twice," "sometimes," "often," and "very often." The inability to meaningfully distinguish between response options independently undermines measurement reliability (Hawthorne, Mouthaan, Forbes, & Novaco, 2006). Therefore, before fielding the two SEQ versions to our sample of 204 soldiers, we simplified the preamble to read "At work, have any of these happened to you in the last year? Someone . . ." followed by the list of SEQ behaviors. Response options were reduced to "never," "once," and "more than once." Other SEQ versions have used these response options.

Because the Department of Defense now uses the SHCore exclusively, we present findings only for the 12-item SHCore and its 16-item plain language counterpart (SHCore-PL; see Table A-1 in the Appendix). The SHCore-PL had a Flesch-Kincaide reading grade level of 2.3.[1]

Problem drinking. We used the TWEAK's "hold" version (Russell et al., 1994) to assess problem drinking. The TWEAK is a 5-item test originally developed to screen for risky drinking during pregnancy, but it also has excellent psychometric properties in men. It includes three of the CAGE (Mayfield, McLeod, & Hall, 1974) alcohol screening questions and also asks about respondents' alcohol tolerance (i.e., how much they can "hold") and blackouts. The TWEAK has a reading grade level of 3.8.

Analysis

Scores for the SHCore and SHCore-PL were calculated by summing respondents' answers to the relevant items. The TWEAK was scored according to its published algorithm (Russell et al., 1994). Analyses were conducted for respondents overall and for subgroups defined by education (with vs. without some college experience) and gender. All reported p values are two-tailed.

Reliability. We followed Murphy and Davidshofer's (1998, p. 143) conventions for interpreting reliability coefficients: .95 indicates that measurement error has "virtually no effect" on test score variance; .90 reflects high to moderate reliability; .75, moderate to low reliability; .65, low reliability; and .50, "true scores and error have equal effects on test scores." Reliabilities below .50 indicate that error accounts for more test score variance than do true score differences. For all measures, we used Cronbach's alpha to assess internal consistency and Pearson's correlation coefficient to assess 1-month test–retest reliability; we also report the mixed model intraclass correlation coefficient (ICC) between tests and retests. For the sexual harassment measures, we used Pearson's correlation coefficient to assess immediate and 1-month alternate-forms reliability, with the SHCore and SHCore-PL serving as each other's alternate form. Defined subgroups' internal consistency and test–retest and alternate-forms reliabilities were compared by applying Fisher's z transformation to each subgroup's correlation and doing a z test on the transformed scale.

Case concordance (kappa). Not all behaviors on the two SHCore versions necessarily meet legal thresholds for sexual harassment. However, we followed common research practice and classified participants as sexual harassment cases if they responded "once" or "more than once" to any test item. Without assigning gold standard status to either test version, we used kappa (κ) to compare case agreement overall and for subgroups defined by education and gender. We used z tests to compare κ across subgroups.

RESULTS

Sociodemographic Characteristics

The education category was missing for two participants and the gender category, for six participants. The sample's mean age was 23.5 years ($SD = 5$). On average, those with college experience were 3.0 years older than those without college experience ($p < .001$), and women were 1.4 years older than men ($p = .04$). A total of 47% of men and 50% of women reported some college experience, $\chi^2 = 0.06$, $N = 198$, $df = 1$, $p = .81$. The remaining sociodemographic characteristics are presented in Table 1. Except for age

TABLE 1 Sociodemographic Characteristics Overall and by Subgroup, Reported as Percentage (%) with the Characteristic

		College experience		Gender	
Characteristic	Over all ($N = 204$)	None ($n = 105$)	Some ($n = 97$)	Male ($n = 108$)	Female ($n = 90$)
Male gender	54.5	55.9	53.1	100	0
Race/ethnicity					
White	50.0	52.4	48.5	54.6	46.7
African American or Black	28.9	31.4	26.8	25.9	31.1
Hispanic	9.3	8.6	10.3	9.3	10.0
Other	12.2	8.6	14.4	11.1	12.2
Highest educational achievement					
Less than 12 years	0.5	1.0	0.0	0.9	0
GED or other High school equivalency	4.0	7.6	0.0	1.9	6.7
High school diploma	47.0	91.4	0.0	50.0	43.3
Less than 2 years of college credit	35.9	0.0	74.2	33.3	38.9
2–4 years of college credit	11.1	0.0	22.6	12.1	10.0
At least some graduate school credit	1.5	0.0	3.1	1.9	1.1
Paygrade					
E1–E2	6.6	6.6	5.2	4.7	8.9
E3	32.8	37.1	28.9	28.7	37.8
E4	52.0	53.3	50.5	58.3	44.4
E5	8.6	1.9	15.5***	8.3	8.9

Notes. Education category was missing for two participants; gender was missing for six participants. GED = general equivalency diploma.

*** $p < .001$ for those without college experience compared to those with college experience.

and paygrade, sociodemographic characteristics did not differ significantly by college experience or gender.

Reliability

SHCore. Table 2 shows reliability estimates and case prevalence for the SHCore. Contrary to expectations, internal consistency did not differ significantly across subgroups. However, compared to those with some college experience, soldiers without college experience demonstrated significantly poorer temporal stability ($z = 2.23$, $p = .01$) and immediate alternate-forms reliability ($z = 2.07$, $p = .02$).

Error accounted for more of the variance in men's SHCore responses over time than did true score differences. Compared to women, men demonstrated substantially poorer temporal stability ($z = -2.15$, $p = .02$), immediate alternate-forms reliability ($z = -2.76$, $p = .003$), and 1-month alternate-forms reliability when the Time 2 SHCore was compared to the Time 1 SHCore-PL ($z = -3.04$, $p = .001$).

SHCore-PL. The SHCore-PL's internal consistency was similar to the SHCore's and did not differ across subgroups (see Table 2). However, in contrast to the SHCore, the SHCore-PL's temporal stability did not differ significantly for soldiers with and without college experience ($z = 1.09$, $p = .17$). Although men's temporal stability was somewhat improved using the SHCore-PL, their responses remained significantly less stable than women's ($z_r = -2.27$, $p_r = .01$; $z_{ICC} = -2.33$, $p_{ICC} = .01$), and error continued to account for half of the variance in their test scores

Kappa. Case agreement did not differ by college experience, but men demonstrated substantially poorer case agreement than women ($z = 5.89$, $p < .001$).

Post Hoc, Exploratory Analysis

To further explore the striking gender difference in reliability, we created four substrata defined by college experience and gender and then compared reliability parameters across them (see Table 3). Because within-stratum numbers were small, there were few statistically significant results. Even so, men without college experience had strikingly poorer SHCore test–retest reliabilities and ICCs than any other group. For men, the SHCore-PL's temporal stability relative to the SHCore's depended on college experience: For men without college experience, the SHCore-PL's temporal stability was qualitatively better; for men with college experience, it was qualitatively worse. For women, the SHCore-PL yielded slightly better reliability parameters than the SHCore regardless of college experience.

TABLE 2 SHCore and SHCore-PL Reliability Estimates and Sexual Harassment Case Prevalence (%) Overall and by Subgroup

	Reliability estimates									
	SHCore				SHCore-PL					
	Internal consistency	1-month test–retest[a]		Alternate forms[a],[b]	Internal consistency	1-month test–retest[a]		Sexual harassment case prevalence		Case agreement
Sample	α	r	ICC	r	α	r	ICC	SHCore	SHCore-PL	κ
Overall (N = 204)	.85	.70	.70	.89/.72/.70	.87	.73	.73	59.8	65.2	.80
By education										
Without college (n = 105)	.85	.57*	.56*	.86*/.68/.61	.88	.69	.67	57.1	62.9	.80
With college (n = 97)	.85	.81	.81	.92/.79/.79	.86	.79	.76	63.9	69.1	.79
By gender										
Male (n = 108)	.85	.40†	.39†	.83†/.45/.37†	.86	.49†	.46†	48.1†	55.5†	.71†
Female (n = 90)	.83	.72	.72	.92/.72/.79	.86	.78	.77	75.6	77.7	.94

Notes. Education category was missing for two participants; gender was missing for six participants. SHCore = Sexual Harassment Core Measure; SHCore-PL = Sexual Harassment Core Measure, plain language counterpart; ICC = intraclass correlation coefficient.

[a]Results are based on 86–89 respondents (39 without college education, 50 with college education 39 men, 47 women). [b]Correlations are presented in this order: SHCore with SHCore-PL, both taken at Time 1/SHCore taken at Time 1 with SHCore-PL 1 month later/SHCore-PL taken at Time 1 with SHCore 1 month later.

*$p \leq .05$ for those without college experience compared to those with college experience.

†$p < .05$ for men compared to women.

TABLE 3 SHCore and SHCore-PL Test–Retest Reliability and Case Agreement After Stratification by Education and Gender

	Reliability estimates					
	1-month test–retest					
	SHCore		SHCore-PL		Alternate forms[a]	Case agreement[b]
Stratum	r	ICC	r	ICC	r	κ
Men						
Without college experience ($n = 19$)	.24*	.21*	.53	.52	.80/.48/.25	.76
With college experience ($n = 20$)	.74	.74	.49	.40	.87/.49/.66	.65
Women						
Without college experience ($n = 17$)	.64	.63	.78	.67	.91/.62/.78	.90[†]
With college experience ($n = 26$)	.77	.77	.81	.81	.93/.77/.81	1.00

Notes. Education category was missing for two participants; gender was missing for six participants. SHCore = Sexual Harassment Core Measure; SHCore-PL = Sexual Harassment Core Measure, plain language counterpart; ICC = intraclass correlation coefficient.

[a]Correlations are presented in this order: SHCore with SHCore-PL, both at Time 1/SHCore at Time 1 with SHCore-PL 1 month later/SHCore-PL at Time 1 with SHCore 1 month later. [b]Results are based on the full sample of 57 men without college experience, 51 men with college experience, 45 women without college experience, and 45 women with college experience.

*$p \leq .05$ comparing men with and without college experience

[†]$p < .05$ comparing women with and without college experience.

TWEAK

As is often seen in brief screening tests designed to maximize criterion-related validity, the TWEAK's internal consistency was low (.38–.46); however, it did not differ significantly by education ($z = 0.16$, $p = .44$) or gender ($z = 0.44$, $p = .33$). One-month test–retest reliabilities and ICCs were moderate (.77–.86) and also did not differ significantly by education ($z_r = 1.00$, $p_r = .16$; $z_{ICC} = 1.06$, $p_{ICC} = .14$) or gender ($z_r = 0.14$, $p_r = .44$; $z_{ICC} = 0.40$, $p_{ICC} = .35$).

DISCUSSION

The military's "gold standard" for assessing sexual harassment performed well in the population for which it was designed: women and individuals with college experience. Most U.S. troops, however, are males without college experience. Among this population, we identified substantial reliability problems. Particularly for men without college experience, more variance in test scores over time was explained by error than by true test score differences. Consequently, the SHCore may not be the ideal instrument for monitoring changes in sexual harassment for most U.S. troops. Claims that sexual harassment prevalence has been declining in the armed forces based on responses to the SHCore (Lipari & Lancaster, 2003) should be viewed cautiously.

Because most of the SEQ's psychometric development has excluded men, it is perhaps not surprising that the instrument does not perform as well in them as in women. However, emerging data using other sexual harassment measures suggest that men sexually harassed in the military are at least as adversely impacted by such experiences as women, if not more so (Vogt, Pless, King, & King, 2005). Inaccurate accounting of men's experiences, especially when it results in undercounts, could lead policymakers and health care workers to minimize the threats sexual harassment might pose for men and divert resources to other, less urgent problems. Therefore, as with women, men's military sexual harassment experiences need to be quantified as accurately as possible.

Writing tests to a population's average reading level may overshoot the reading abilities of many, which in turn could lead to satisficed or inaccurate responses. Even though military recruits on average read at the 11th-grade level and the SHCore reads at the 9th-grade level, our focus groups showed that several participants had problems understanding it. In the present sample, the SHCore's test–retest reliability and alternate-forms reliability were also substantially poorer in soldiers without college experience compared to those with college experience. Because our sample actually had more college experience than U.S. troops at large, it seems likely that these problems would be amplified in the larger military population. Likewise, because the general U.S. population tends to have lower literacy skills than persons in the military, comprehension problems might also affect civilian SEQ versions.

Although we created the SHCore-PL in hopes of reducing cognitive burden for soldiers with lower reading aptitudes, results using the SHCore-PL were mixed. It performed very well in women, regardless of college experience, and improved test performance for men without college experience as expected; however, it actually degraded performance for men with college experience. Schuman and Presser (1996, p. 6) speculated that when asked survey questions, well-educated individuals might be particularly sensitive to "precise verbal distinctions." As suggested by our focus groups, by simplifying the SHCore we may have discarded nuances important to the responses of college educated men. Furthermore, despite the SHCore-PL's better performance in men without college experience, error still accounted for almost as much of the variance in their SHCore-PL scores as was accounted for by true test score differences. In contrast, the TWEAK, which is written at the fourth-grade level, showed no evidence of unreliability by education or gender. This suggests that the problems we identified in the SHCore/SHCore-PL were specific to those measures and not a general tendency of our sample to satisfice.

Although provocative, the present study has several limitations. First, the findings were based on a convenience sample. Although our enrollment method has been used in other military studies and is thought to generate reasonably representative samples from any given military facility (Rosen & Martin, 1998; Wolfe, Brown, & Kelley, 1993), the findings may not generalize to soldiers stationed at other locations or to other military branches. In addition, our participants were more likely to have had college experience than the military at large.

Second, actual changes in sexual harassment events could have given an appearance of temporal unreliability in soldiers' responses between the first and second tests. Reactivity, in which answering questions induces changes in respondents' perceptions (Carmines & Zeller, 1979), and priming effects, which trigger test takers to remember additional events after their first sitting, could also have led to spuriously low test–retest reliability estimates. However, all of these effects should have resulted in soldiers reporting more events on the second test compared to the first one. Among respondents with discordant test results, half to four fifths indicated no sexual harassment experiences on retesting but some during the original assessment.

Third, satisficing can be measured directly only by comparing participants' answers to their actual experiences. Because this is usually unfeasible, most investigators rely on indirect evidence, such as reliability measures, to infer the presence of satisficing (Krosnick et al., 2002). However, satisficing is not the only reason why tests prove to be unreliable.

Fourth and most important, we do not know whether the unreliability we documented in men and soldiers without college experience resulted in biased or unbiased test error. As long as very large sample sizes are used, only biased error would meaningfully influence sexual harassment prevalence or effect size estimates. However, satisficing that leads to biased error (e.g., systematic under- or overcounting) cannot be overcome with larger sample sizes. Furthermore, data collected from smaller samples would continue to be at risk for misinterpretation. Although it seems inefficient and undesirable to knowingly use a survey instrument that underperforms in most U.S. troops, our data are too preliminary to recommend abandoning the SHCore. We do, however, encourage replication in larger, more representative samples. Comprehensive clinical and cognitive interviews might also clarify whether the SHCore systematically over- or underestimates men's sexual harassment experiences. If systematic bias is identified, perhaps the armed forces could consider creating a military-specific measure of sexual harassment that follows more usual survey development (i.e., item generation from key informants and focus groups, psychometric analysis of the entire item pool, and cognitive interviews and reliability testing of the resulting instrument).

The military independently represents a large segment of the U.S. population; however, these results carry implications beyond the armed forces and even beyond the field of sexual harassment. Specifically, our findings highlight problems that can arise when measures developed in one population are applied to a new population without adequate pretesting. Feedback, in the form of focus groups or cognitive interviews, must be elicited from members of the new population to ensure that the measure remains readable, applicable, and consistently and correctly interpreted. When feedback cannot be obtained, post hoc reliability assessments across selected subgroups may help identify potential problems. Unfortunately, although Cronbach's alpha is easily obtained and popular in social science research, correlated errors tend to inflate it (Green, 2003). Thus, it may not be terribly useful for identifying problems related to satisficing. In the present study, Cronbach's alpha seemed a less sensitive indicator of potential satisficing than test–retest and alternate-forms reliability. We encourage researchers to consider risks for satisficing (e.g., by attending to reading level and saliency) when developing new survey tools and when applying preexisting measures to new populations. These concerns are particularly acute when the topic is socially important and carries policy implications.

NOTE

1. The 12-item SHCore had a correlation of .96 with the Department of Defense's original SEQ version. The 16-item SHCore-PL had a correlation of .96 with the 31-item plain language SEQ version. Analyses of the Department of Defense's full SEQ version and its plain language counterpart are available on request and essentially mirror the results reported here.

REFERENCES

Antecol, H., & Cobb-Clark, D. (2006). The sexual harassment of female active-duty personnel: Effects on job satisfaction and intentions to remain in the military. *Journal of Economic Behavior & Organization, 61*, 55.

Bastian, L., Lancaster, A., & Reyst, H. (1996). *Department of Defense 1995 Sexual Harassment Survey* (Report No. 96-014). Arlington, VA: Defense Manpower Data Center.

Berdahl, J., Magley, V., & Waldo, C. (1996). The sexual harassment of men? Exploring the concept with theory and data. *Psychology of Women Quarterly, 20*, 527–547.

Carmines, E., & Zeller, R. (1979). *Reliability and validity assessment* (Vol. 17). Newbury Park, CA: Sage.

Culbertson, A., Rosenfeld, P., & Newell, C. (1993). *Sexual harassment in the active-duty Navy. Findings from the 1991 Navy-wide survey* (Publication No. TR-94-2). San Diego, CA: Navy Personnel Research and Development Center.

Department of Defense. (2004). *Office of the Undersecretary of Defense, Personnel and Readiness: Population representation in the military services: Fiscal year 2002*. Washington, DC: Department of Defence.

Doak, C., Doak, L., & Root, J. (1996). *Teaching patients with low literacy skills*. Philadelphia, PA: Lippincott.

Fitzgerald, L., Gelfand, M., & Drasgow, F. (1995). Measuring sexual harassment: Theoretical and psychometric advances. *Basic and Applied Social Psychology, 17*, 425–445.

Fitzgerald, L., Magley, V., Drasgow, F., & Waldo, C. (1999). Measuring sexual harassment in the military: The Sexual Experiences Questionnaire (SEQ-DoD). *Military Psychology, 11*, 243–263.

Fitzgerald, L., Shullman, S., Bailey, N., Richards, M., Swecker, J., Gold, Y., ... Weitzman, L. (1988). The incidence and dimensions of sexual harassment in academia and the work place. *Journal of Vocational Behavior,, ,32*, 152–175.

Gelfand, M., Fitzgerald, L., & Drasgow, F. (1995). The structure of sexual harassment: A confirmatory analysis across cultures and settings. *Journal of Vocational Behavior, 47*, 164–177.

Green, S. B. (2003). A coefficient alpha for test-retest data. *Psychological Methods, 8*, 88–101.

Guyatt, G. H., Walter, S., & Norman, G. (1987). Measuring change over time: Assessing the usefulness of evaluative instruments. *Journal of Chronic Disease, 40*, 171–178.

Hawthorne, G., Mouthaan, J., Forbes, D., & Novaco, R. W. (2006). Response categories and anger measurement: Do fewer categories result in poorer measurement? Development of the DAR5. *Social Psychiatry and Psychiatric Epidemiology, 41*, 164–172.

Kang, H., Dalager, N., Mahan, C., & Ishii, E. (2005). The role of sexual assault on the risk of PTSD among Gulf War veterans. *Annals of Epidemiology, 15*, 191–195.

Kincaid, J., Fishburne, R., Rogers, R., & Chisson, B. (1975). *Derivation of new readability formulas (Automated Readability Index, Fog count, and Flesch Reading Ease Formula) for Navy enlisted personnel* (Research Branch Report No. 8-75). Millington: Naval Technical Training, U.S. Naval Air Station, Memphis, TN.

Krosnick, J. A. (1991). Response strategies for coping with the cognitive demands of attitude measures in surveys. *Applied Cognitive Psychology, 5*, 213–236.

Krosnick, J. A., Holbrook, A. L , Berent, M. K., Carson, R. T., Hanemann, W., Kopp, R. J., ... Conaway, M. (2002). The impact of "no opinion" response options on data quality: Non-attitude reduction or an invitation to satisfice? *Public Opinion Quarterly, 66*, 371–403.

Lam, T. C., & Bengo, P. (2003). A comparison of three retrospective self-reporting methods of measuring change in instructional practice. *American Journal of Evaluation, 24*, 65–80.

Lipari, R., & Lancaster, A. (2003). *Armed Forces 2002 Sexual Harassment Survey* (No. 2003-026). Arlington, VA: Defense Manpower Data Center, Department of Defense.

Mayfield, D., McLeod, G., & Hall, P. (1974). The CAGE questionnaire: Validation of an alcoholism screening instrument. *American Journal of Psychiatry, 131*, 1121–1123.

Murphy, K. R., & Davidshofer, C. O. (1998). Using and interpreting information about test reliability. In K. R. Murphy & C. O. Davidshofer (Eds.), *Psychological testing: Principles and applications* (4th ed., pp. 127–145). Upper Saddle River, NJ: Prentice Hall.

Pryor, J. (1995). The psychosocial impact of sexual harassment on women in the U.S. military. *Basic and Applied Social Psychology, 17*, 581–603.

Rosen, L., & Martin, L. (1998). Childhood maltreatment history as a risk factor for sexual harassment among US Army soldiers. *Violence & Victims, 13*, 269–286.

Russell, M., Martier, S., Sokol, R., Mudar, P., Bottoms, S., Jacobson, S., & Jacobsen, J. (1994). Screening for pregnancy risk-drinking. *Alcoholism: Clinical and Experimental Research, 18*, 1156–1161.

Schuman, H., & Presser, S. (1996). *Questions and answers in attitude surveys: Experiments on question form, wording, and context*. Thousand Oaks, CA: Sage.

Stark, S., Chernyshenko, O. S., Lancaster, A. R., Drasgow, F., & Fitzgerald, L. F. (2002). Toward standardized measurement of sexual harassment: Shortening the SEQ-DoD using item response theory. *Military Psychology, 14*, 49–72.

Vogt, D., Pless, A. P., King, L. A., & King, D. W. (2005). Deployment stressors, gender, and mental health outcomes among Gulf War I veterans. *Journal of Traumatic Stress, 18*, 115–127.

Waldo, C., Berdahl, J., & Fitzgerald, L. (1998). Are men sexually harassed? If so, by whom? *Law and Human Behavior, 22*, 59–79.

Wolfe, J., Brown, P., & Kelley, J. (1993). Reassessing war stress: Exposure and the Persian Gulf War. *Journal of Social Issues, 49*, 15–31.

APPENDIX

TABLE A-1 Item Content of the SHCore and Its Plain Language Counterpart (SHCore-PL)

SHCore items		Corresponding plain language items (SHCore-PL)	
1	Told sexual stories or jokes that were offensive to you?	1	Told sexual stories or jokes that were offensive to you?
2	Made unwelcome attempts to draw you into a discussion of sexual matters (for example, attempted to discuss or comment on your sex life)?	2′	Tried to talk "sexy" with you when you didn't want to?
3	Made offensive remarks about your appearance, body, or sexual activities?	3a′	Made crude comments about your body?
		3b′	Made crude comments about how you looked?
4	Made gestures or used body language of a sexual nature which embarrassed or offended you?	4a′	Made crude sexual gestures that made you blush?
		4b′	Acted out sex acts in front of you?

(Continued)

TABLE A-1 (Continued)

SHCore items		Corresponding plain language items (SHCore-PL)	
5	Made unwanted attempts to establish a romantic sexual relationship with you despite your efforts to discourage it?	5a′	Kept trying to go out with me, even after I said I didn't want to?
		5b′	Kept trying to have a sexual romance with me, even though I said I wasn't interested?
6	Continued to ask you for dates, drinks, dinner, etc., even though you said "No"?	6′[a]	Kept asking you to go out with him/her even after you said you didn't want to?
7	Made you feel like you were being bribed with some sort of reward or special treatment to engage in sexual behavior?	7′	Hinted that you would be treated extra nice if you had sex with him or her?
8	Made you feel threatened with some sort of retaliation for not being sexually cooperative (for example, by mentioning an upcoming review)?	8′	Said you'd get a bad review if you didn't have sex with him/her?
9	Touched you in a way that made you feel uncomfortable?	9′	Touched you in a sexual way?
10	Made unwanted attempts to stroke, fondle, or kiss you?	10a′	Tried to stroke you when you didn't want him/her to?
		10b′	Tried to fondle you when you didn't want him/her to?
		10c′	Tried to kiss you when you didn't want him/her to?
11	Treated you badly for refusing to have sex?	11′	Treated you badly after you said you wouldn't have sex with him/her?
12	Implied faster promotions or better treatment if you were sexually cooperative?	12′	Offered you a promotion in exchange for sex?

Notes. SHCore = Sexual Harassment Core Measure; SHCore-PL = Sexual Harassment Core Measure, plain language counterpart.

[a]This item was omitted from the SHCore-PL because it was nearly identical to item 5a′.

Veterans Health Administration Mental Health Treatment Settings of Patients Who Report Military Sexual Trauma

COURTNEY VALDEZ, PhD, RACHEL KIMERLING, PhD,
JENNY K. HYUN, PhD, HANNA F. MARK, BA,
MEGHAN SAWEIKIS, MS, and JOANNE PAVAO, MPH

National Center for Posttraumatic Stress Disorder, VA Palo Alto Health Care System, Palo Alto, California, USA

The comprehensive Veterans Health Administration (VHA) policies on military sexual trauma (MST) include provider education and training at each VHA facility. No published data exist that indicate the settings in which VHA mental health patients with MST are treated. Such information could help set priorities for targeted MST-related education and training. The major aim of this article was to describe the VHA mental health outpatient settings in which patients with MST are most likely to be treated. National data from 79,903 female and 889,998 male veteran patients with at least one face-to-face outpatient mental health encounter at any VHA facility in fiscal year 2008 were analyzed. Among all veterans in VHA outpatient mental health care, 35.8% of women and 2.4% of men reported MST. The proportion of MST-positive patients ranged from 25.9% to 81.0% of women and from 1.5% to 56.1% of men

---

Funding was provided in part by the Health Services Research and Development Service, U.S. Department of Veterans Affairs IAE 05–291. The funding source had no role in the study design; data collection, analysis, or interpretation; manuscript preparation; or decision to publish the manuscript. The views expressed in this article are those of the authors and do not necessarily reflect the position or policy of the Department of Veterans Affairs. The authors declare no conflicts of interest or financial relationships related to this research. The authors would like to acknowledge Deborah Nazarian, PhD, and Gloria G. Maramba, PhD, for their consultation.

across 9 major clinic setting categories. Proportions of women with MST were substantial across specialty MST clinics, specialty posttraumatic stress disorder clinics, psychosocial rehabilitation, and substance use disorder clinics, reflecting a wide range of settings. These settings should be prioritized for MST-related provider education and training. By contrast, male MST patients represented only a small proportion of patients in all clinics, with the exception of MST specialty clinics. Tailored conceptualizations of trauma-informed care are proposed for settings that encounter MST patients, even if these settings do not directly focus on the treatment of traumatic stress.

Military sexual trauma (MST) is the term used by the Department of Veterans Affairs to refer to sexual assault and to repeated, threatening sexual harassment occurring during military service. Recent estimates reveal that 21.5% of female and 1.1% of male veterans presenting to the Veterans Health Administration (VHA) for care report a history of MST and that such experiences are associated with substantially elevated rates of mental health conditions (Kimerling, Gima, Smith, Street, & Frayne, 2007). Because MST is a stressor rather than a mental health diagnosis, VHA policies around MST focus on detection and access to care for the wide range of conditions associated with MST. Subsequent mental health treatment, when indicated, can be provided in a variety of settings based on each individual's specific symptoms or diagnosis. Although not all patients who report a history of MST will need or want mental health treatment, like other potentially traumatic stressors MST has been shown to lead to the development of posttraumatic stress disorder (PTSD; Kang, Dalager, Mahan, & Ishii, 2005) or to function as one of several life events relevant to the treatment of other mental health conditions, such as depression, anxiety, or substance use disorders (Kimerling et al., 2007; Street, Stafford, Mahan, & Hendricks, 2008). Despite the range of symptoms and diagnoses related to MST, there are little data that describe the VHA mental health settings where MST patients are most likely to receive care.

In both veteran and civilian populations, few individuals disclose experiences of interpersonal violence like sexual trauma unless asked because of factors that may include social stigma and self-blame (Campbell & Raja, 2005: McCauley, Yurk, Jenckes, & Ford, 1998; Rennison, 2002). VHA policy requires universal screening for MST and documentation in the patient's electronic medical record to ensure effective detection (VHA, 2008). At every VHA facility, designated MST coordinators facilitate treatment for sexual trauma upon provider determination of clinical need, and care for all related conditions is delivered free of charge. This care is most often mental health care, and the universal screening program for MST appears to be an effective means of increasing access to mental health services for this population, especially among veterans without prior mental health treatment (Kimerling, Street, Gima, & Smith, 2008). In addition to the universal screening policy, VHA provides MST-related education for mental health professionals and other health care personnel. Identifying where MST patients are overrepresented in VHA outpatient mental health care is a first step in determining high-priority mental health settings to target these MST-related resources and to assess local needs for MST-related training and education.

Highlighting potential clinical issues unique to sexual trauma and relevant to a variety of mental health settings is particularly important because relative to VHA patients who do not report MST, patients with MST demonstrate an increased likelihood of a variety of mental health conditions (Kimerling et al., 2007) treated in a variety of settings. VHA has established specialty MST clinics to address the clinical needs of patients who have experienced MST. However, these clinics cannot be expected to provide the full range of mental health services necessary to treat the wide spectrum of MST-related mental health conditions. Given the finding that PTSD is the most frequent mental health condition associated with MST (Kang et al., 2005; Kimerling et al., 2007; Street et al., 2008), a significant proportion of female and male patients with MST may be treated in VHA's PTSD specialty clinics. Although there is not yet research that has examined the need for or impact of provider training and education on sexual trauma, it is reasonable to assume that providers in trauma-focused settings are among those most familiar with issues related to MST. Therefore, these settings may serve as high-priority targets for MST-related resource and support allocation decisions. Also, providers in these trauma-focused settings could be preliminarily identified as having some local expertise in MST-related care, thereby serving as key individuals in forming networks of care with providers in other mental health settings who are also treating patients with MST.

In addition to PTSD, women and men who have experienced MST are more likely than women and men who do not report MST to be diagnosed with anxiety disorders, depression, dissociative disorders, eating disorders, bipolar disorder, substance use disorders, and personality disorders (Kimerling et al., 2007; Street et al., 2008; Suris & Lind, 2008). Furthermore, MST has been associated with a host of functional impairments (Murdoch, Pryor, Polusny, & Gackstetter, 2007; Suris, Lind, Kashner, & Borman, 2007). Taken together, these studies suggest that awareness of MST-related issues is relevant for a broad range of mental health settings, such as clinics that provide treatments for substance abuse, chronic mental illness, or affective and anxiety disorders. If MST patients are indeed overrepresented in these settings, then these would also be potential targets for MST-related resources and education. In such settings, educational efforts might address basic facts about MST, issues surrounding disclosure of trauma, and/or trauma-related interpersonal and functional challenges.

The major aim of this article is to describe the VHA mental health outpatient settings in which patients who report MST are most likely to be treated. These data will support MST training and education efforts, inform resource allocation decisions, and potentially empower providers to create local networks of MST-related care. We examined national data from VHA electronic medical records for all mental health outpatient services provided to veterans in fiscal year 2008. We explored the settings where mental health patients with MST are most frequently treated by broadly grouping mental health clinics and examining the proportion of patients treated in each setting who report MST. We then determined in which settings patients with a history of MST are overrepresented. Ultimately, any mental health patient with a history of MST would benefit from being served in a setting where providers have the necessary resources, education, and training available to assess and to address their patients' multifaceted needs.

METHOD

Study Design and Population

This is a national, cross-sectional, descriptive study of the 1,017,244 veterans with at least one face-to-face outpatient mental health encounter at a VHA facility between October 1, 2007, and September 30, 2008. Data on MST screening and mental health utilization were abstracted from the electronic medical record. We describe the 95.3% of the total population (969,901 veterans: 79,903 women and 889,998 men) who were screened for MST, excluding the 0.5% (5,419 veterans) who declined screening and the 4.1% (41,924 veterans) who had not yet been screened for MST. Approval for the study was obtained from the Stanford University School of Medicine institutional review board.

Data Sources

We used VHA administrative data sets for fiscal year 2008. MST data are captured in the patient's electronic medical record through the use of a clinical reminder. The VHA's Outpatient Events File provides demographic and clinical encounter information on all VHA outpatients. Each patient encounter with a provider yields a unique record with a primary diagnosis, demographics, a clinic stop code that documents where care was provided, and other clinical information.

Key Variables

VHA uses a clinical reminder in the patient's electronic medical record to screen for MST. The brief screening instrument contains the following items: "While you were in the military: (a) Did you receive uninvited and unwanted sexual attention, such as touching, cornering, pressure for sexual favors, or verbal remarks?; (b) Did someone ever use force or threat of force to have sexual contact with you against your will?" An affirmative response to either question is recorded as a positive experience of MST.

VHA uses clinic stop codes as a means of documenting where care is provided. A modified Delphi consensus approach was used to group stop codes, with classification consensus achieved among four experienced VHA mental health providers representing clinical care, administration, and program evaluation. The 63 outpatient mental health clinic stop codes were categorized into nine non-overlapping groups: (a) specialty MST clinics specifically designed to treat conditions related to MST (clinic stop code 524); (b) specialty PTSD clinics, including services provided by PTSD Clinical Teams and Women's Stress Disorder Treatment Teams (clinic stop codes 516, 525, 540, 542, 561, 562, 580, 581); (c) psychosocial rehabilitation and mental health intensive case management (MHICM) clinics (clinic stop codes 532, 537, 546, 552, 559, 564, 567, 582, 583, 584); (d) specialty substance use disorder treatment clinics, including individual, group, and day program substance abuse settings (clinic stop codes 513, 519, 523, 545, 547, 560); (e) vocational rehabilitation, such as compensated work therapy (clinic stop codes 535, 536, 568, 573, 574, 575); (f) housing support services, such as housing, consultation, and referral services provided through the Health Care for Homeless Veterans and Homeless Chronically Mentally Ill programs (clinic stop codes 522, 528, 529, 530, 590, 591); (g) general mental health settings, such as mental health clinics and individual psychology and psychiatry treatment (clinic stop codes 502, 505, 506, 509, 510, 512, 527, 538, 550, 553, 554, 557, 558, 576, 577, 578, 579, 589); (h) behavioral health clinics, including behavioral medicine and primary care mental health integration programs (clinic stop codes 322 + any 500, 323 + any 500, 531, 533, 534, 563, 565, 566); and (i) returning Operation Enduring Freedom/Operation Iraqi Freedom veteran outreach services (clinic stop codes 571, 572).

Statistical Procedures

To determine the VHA mental health outpatient settings in which patients who report MST are most likely to be treated, we used independent chi-square tests to examine the proportion of MST patients observed in each health clinic setting compared to the proportion of MST patients seen in all other outpatient mental health clinic settings. Analyses were repeated to examine each mental health clinic setting. Veterans were the unit of analysis for all comparisons, but veterans who used multiple clinic types were analyzed in each of the settings they utilized. All analyses were calculated separately by gender. Because of the large sample size, statistically significant differences were tested using a two-sided significance level of $p < .01$. A Bonferroni correction was used for multiple comparisons, resulting in a significance level of $p < .001$.

RESULTS

Among all veterans who used VHA outpatient mental health care, 35.8% of women and 2.4% of men reported a history of MST. Both women and men with MST were more likely to use more than one mental health clinic type as compared to those who have not experienced MST (among women 37.2% versus 24.8%, $\chi^2(1, N = 79{,}903) = 1{,}378.65$, $p < .0001$ and among men 38.8% versus 28.7%, $\chi^2(1, N = 889{,}998) = 1{,}028.34$, $p < .0001$). Among all mental health patients who used multiple clinic types, the majority used only two types (71.5%). Table 1 describes the proportion of patients who reported a history of MST within each VHA outpatient mental health clinic setting, stratified by gender. Specifically, Table 1 reports the total number of mental health patients who used each clinic setting in fiscal year 2008 and the number and percentage of those patients who reported MST. Chi-square statistics reflect the comparisons between the proportion of MST patients observed in each mental health clinic setting and the proportion of MST patients seen in all other outpatient mental health clinic settings. As expected, among women, a significantly larger proportion of patients in MST specialty clinics reported MST as compared to the proportion of patients among all other settings who reported MST: 81.0% vs. 34.2%, $\chi^2(1, N = 79{,}903) = 2{,}565.89$, $p < .0001$. Among women, MST was similarly significantly overrepresented in the following clinic types: specialty PTSD, psychosocial rehabilitation/MHICM, specialty substance use, vocational rehabilitation, and housing support services. Also as expected, among men, a significantly larger proportion of patients in MST specialty clinics reported MST as compared to the proportion of patients among all other settings who reported MST: 56.1% vs. 2.3%, $\chi^2(1, N = 889{,}998) = 15{,}497.89$, $p < .0001$. MST was similarly significantly overrepresented among men in the following clinic types: specialty PTSD, psychosocial rehabilitation/MHICM, specialty substance use, vocational rehabilitation, housing support services, general mental health, and behavioral health. In addition, among both women and men, the proportion of patients who reported MST in Operation Enduring Freedom/Operation Iraqi Freedom outreach clinics was significantly less than the proportion of patients among all other settings who reported MST. Female MST patients represented substantial proportions of the female veterans seen in many clinic settings examined, whereas male

TABLE 1 Proportion of MST+ Veterans in VHA Mental Health Outpatients by Clinic Setting: October 1, 2007–September 30, 2008

	Women				Men			
	Total clinic	MST+			Total clinic	MST+		
Setting	users	n	%	χ^2	users	n	%	χ^2
All mental health settings	79,903	28,610	35.8		889,998	21,538	2.4	
Specialty MST	2,788	2,258	81.0	2,565.89**	1,270	712	56.1	15,497.89**
Specialty PTSD	10,403	5,580	53.6	1,654.66**	138,352	4,168	3.0	243.62**
Psychosocial rehabilitation/ MHICM	2,530	1,114	44.0	76.91**	25,541	1,011	4.0	263.52**
Specialty substance use	6,105	2,633	43.1	154.20**	119,679	3,710	3.1	270.72**
Vocational rehabilitation services	2,857	1,210	42.4	55.24**	37,858	1,302	3.4	173.92**
Housing support services	3,601	1,474	40.9	43.13**	60,978	1,885	3.1	124.92**
General mental health	71,549	25,730	36.0	7.20	754,308	18,930	2.5	168.12**
Behavioral health	9,941	3,530	35.5	0.43	99,788	2,717	2.7	43.63**
OEF/OIF outreach services	2,219	574	25.9	98.08**	18,886	279	1.5	72.62**

Notes: To reduce redundancy, we do not show the proportion of MST patients in all other outpatient mental health clinic settings for each comparison, but these proportions varied between 33.1% and 36.1% among women and 1.9% and 2.4% among men. MST + = number (n) and percentage (%) of veterans who report military sexual trauma (MST) by clinic setting; VHA = Veterans Health Administration; PTSD = posttraumatic stress disorder; MHICM = mental health intensive case management; OEF/OIF = Operation Enduring Freedom/Operation Iraqi Freedom.
** $p < .0001$.

MST patients represented only a small proportion of patients in all clinics in which they were seen, with the exception of MST specialty clinics.

DISCUSSION

MST is common among VHA mental health outpatients. More than one third of women and 2.4% of men seen in outpatient mental health settings report a history of MST. Our results indicate that across many settings, VHA mental health providers, especially those who treat women, are quite likely to encounter patients who have experienced MST. Not surprisingly, the highest proportions of female and male MST patients were treated in

MST specialty clinics. We also found that although MST patients were over-represented in specialty PTSD treatment settings, substantial proportions of MST patients were also found across a broad range of other clinical settings. Clinically significant effects were observed for female patients in psychosocial rehabilitation/MHICM and substance use treatment settings. These clinics appear to treat many female patients with MST histories and thus are appropriate priorities for MST-related resources and educational efforts. Training levels vary across clinical settings at each VHA facility, but these data indicate that national priorities for MST education should be defined broadly and tailored to the scope of care appropriate to settings that address a range of clinical conditions and functional domains.

Overall, our findings suggest that mental health providers who treat female veterans, even if they work in settings that do not traditionally incorporate interventions focused on traumatic stress, may encounter issues related to MST and should be aware that they are working with sexually traumatized populations. Therefore, in all mental health settings, training in how to respond to sexual trauma disclosure is an important first step. In their sample of primarily African American female veterans, Campbell and Raja (2005) found that provider response to sexual trauma disclosure had a significant impact; after disclosure, most women in this sample retrospectively reported experiences of secondary victimization and victim-blaming behaviors by military providers. Research also suggests that many providers are hesitant to broach areas in which they feel underqualified, such as interpersonal violence, perhaps for fear of giving the "wrong" response to patients (Markoff, Finkelstein, Kammerer, Kreiner, & Prost, 2005; Sugg & Inui, 1992). However, recent evidence from male and female veterans with PTSD in VHA health care suggests that despite mixed perceptions of positive and negative responses to trauma disclosure from providers, the majority of patients reported that they were glad that they had disclosed (Leibowitz, Jeffreys, Copeland, & Noel, 2008). Although not specific to sexual trauma disclosure, this finding was true regardless of the type of provider to whom the disclosure was made, suggesting that providers need not be trauma specialists in order to approach these topics with patients.

Other settings are likely to benefit from education regarding the impact of MST on functional outcomes and from training that would familiarize providers with common related interpersonal and functional difficulties. Providers in these settings might encounter patients with MST who struggle with trust, safety, and intimacy in relationships both with their providers and with others in their social networks (Pearlman & Courtois, 2005). Because MST is an experience that occurs within a work and/or home environment, veterans reporting MST may be particularly impacted in their attempts to succeed in future vocational and housing opportunities. Providers in settings who work with patients to prepare for job interviews or negotiate housing arrangements and who possess MST-related education and training are likely to be prepared to address related interpersonal and functional difficulties and/or to recognize opportunities to make referrals for trauma-focused care.

VHA's comprehensive policies for the detection and treatment of sexual trauma (VHA, 2005, 2008) present a unique opportunity to consider the valuable role that MST experts and trauma specialists play in using their skills to promote effective treatment for MST across the wide range of mental health settings used by MST patients. Clinicians in trauma-focused settings who possess specialized expertise in sexual trauma are qualified to serve as locally based experts or consultants. The informal development of consultation groups or relationships with providers across clinic settings has the potential to broaden the settings in which MST-related issues are addressed or to increase providers' comfort in addressing these issues. Providers in trauma-focused settings who have expertise in trauma-informed care and knowledge about the role of sexual trauma in psychological and behavioral functioning, such as facility MST coordinators, are valuable assets within and across mental health settings. Given our findings that significant proportions of mental health outpatients with MST are seen across multiple treatment settings, these specialists should be empowered to develop care coordination and consultation networks with other providers who are less familiar with trauma-informed care.

Lastly, it is important to consider the impact of gender on both mental health diagnosis and mental health care utilization, especially in sexually traumatized populations (Street, Kimerling, Bell, & Pavao, 2011; Zinzow, Grubaugh, Frueh, & Magruder, 2008). Compared with their male counterparts, female VHA mental health outpatients report markedly higher rates of MST. Although not every woman veteran in outpatient mental health care has reported MST, given that more than one third of women in VHA mental health care have reported MST, all VHA clinicians who see women must have some knowledge of MST. For these clinicians it can be helpful at the very least to consider the ways in which gender role socialization influences patient perceptions of interpersonal safety. For example, women who have experienced interpersonal violence have been shown to report more fear of bodily injury than have men (Tjaden & Thoennes, 2000), which may have a resulting impact on their perceptions of interpersonal safety. The issue of safety presents itself in a variety of settings, such as when patients express a preference for a clinician of a particular gender. This preference may be due in part to fear of proximity to an individual of the same gender as their perpetrator(s) (Street et al., 2011). Therefore, providers in all settings also should be educated in the current best practice of giving patients a choice in provider gender (Street et al., 2011).

Although proportions of male veterans who report MST are substantially larger in mental health settings compared to the overall 1% prevalence in VHA (Kimerling et al., 2007), our findings show that they are still a relative minority in mental health settings outside of MST specialty clinics. Some evidence suggests that males are more vulnerable than females to the negative mental health consequences of MST (Street, Gradus, Stafford, & Kelly, 2007). Providers across settings are thus called to be attuned to this minority group and not to overlook the role of MST in the mental health care of male veterans. Relative to women, men may be less likely to disclose MST—possibly because of increased stigma related to fear of disbelief or stereotyping from others (Street et al., 2011). At a minimum, education about effective and appropriate responses to sexual trauma disclosure should be offered across mental health settings. Advanced provider training in clinical interventions that seek to support the full range of emotional expression without fear of stigmatization (Street et al., 2011) should be prioritized in some mental health treatment settings with higher relative proportions of male patients with MST.

This study has some limitations. First, the mental health treatment settings described here reflect the broad range of settings used by MST patients but do not necessarily indicate that MST was the presenting problem or primary focus of treatment. We propose that proportions of MST-positive patients in MST specialty clinics are not 100% because these clinics now provide resources for the treatment of other forms of sexual trauma over the life span. These clinics may also address the consequences of stressors such as child sexual abuse or intimate partner violence. Second, we decided to look at patients with MST who were currently receiving services within VHA mental health care as a way to focus recommendations for education, training, and resource support for providers and leadership. This does not allow us to generalize the findings to all MST-positive veterans inside or outside of VHA health care. However, because VHA is the largest health care system in the country, our ability to look at the entire VHA mental health population does offer other large health care systems a potential method for identifying high-priority settings where providers are likely to benefit from education, training, and consultation targeted to sexual trauma. Our conservative statistical approach with our large national sample provided an opportunity to differentiate between statistically significant and clinically significant effects, so that these results generalize across VHA mental health care and provide basic information with which facility leaders can make their own training and educational decisions. Lastly, we were unable to assess for the kind of training already received across VHA mental health settings or to assess where there may be an unmet education and training need. Ultimately, education and training decisions are most often made at the facility level. Yet these results do provide policymakers with basic data that can guide VHA's comprehensive and unprecedented commitment to offering necessary provider education and training related to sexual trauma.

Overall, our results indicate that VHA mental health patients with MST are seen outside of trauma-focused treatment settings, and thus providers should be aware of MST-related issues in a wide range of settings. Education and training efforts, although typically implemented locally, can be prioritized based on the likelihood of encountering patients with MST in a given mental health setting and can focus on clinical issues related to sexual trauma across a wide range of settings. Mental health clinicians in trauma-focused treatment settings and in settings that treat women are likely to encounter patients with MST. These settings should be targeted for training and education opportunities in issues related to the disclosure and care of sexual trauma, the principles of trauma-informed care, and the creation of local care coordination and consultation networks. Providers in settings with relatively high rates of MST among their male patients should be offered education that will help address the potential impact of stigma in this population. Future research should focus on better understanding the factors that might affect treatment access and use among patients who report a history of MST (e.g., proximity and access to VHA, patient comfort with mental health care) and organizational or educational interventions to promote awareness of trauma-informed care. Research targeting specific clinical settings may also offer conclusions that could guide specific educational efforts. Building on these data, which focus on the mental health treatment settings of patients who report MST, targeted investigations of provider practices and needs within these settings also are likely to inform educational efforts. Moreover, this current study focused exclusively on mental health patients in VHA and made comparisons within this subgroup as a way to guide mental health education and training efforts. Although it was beyond the scope of the current investigation to look at MST-positive veterans outside of mental health settings, a future paper examining the care patterns of MST patients in physical health care likely would be beneficial and may inform educational and training efforts in non–mental health settings.

REFERENCES

Campbell, R., & Raja, S. (2005). The sexual assault and secondary victimization of female veterans: Help-seeking experiences with military and civilian social systems. *Psychology of Women Quarterly*, *29*(1), 97–106.

Kang, H., Dalager, N., Mahan, C., & Ishii, E. (2005). The role of sexual assault on the risk of PTSD among Gulf War veterans. *Annals of Epidemiology*, *15*(3), 191–195.

Kimerling, R., Gima, K., Smith, M. W., Street, A. E., & Frayne, S. (2007). The Veterans Health Administration and military sexual trauma. *American Journal of Public Health*, *97*, 2160–2166.

Kimerling, R., Street, A. E., Gima, K., & Smith, M. W. (2008). Evaluation of universal screening for military-related sexual trauma. *Psychiatric Services*, *59*, 635–640.

Leibowitz, R. Q., Jeffreys, M. D., Copeland, L. A., & Noel, P. H. (2008). Veterans' disclosure of trauma to healthcare providers. *General Hospital Psychiatry*, *30*(2), 100–103.

Markoff, L., Finkelstein, N., Kammerer, N., Kreiner, P., & Prost, C. (2005). Relational systems change: Implementing a model of change in integrating services for women with substance abuse and mental health disorders and histories of trauma. *Journal of Behavioral Health Services & Research*, *32*(2), 227–240.

McCauley, J., Yurk, R. A., Jenckes, M. W., & Ford, D. E. (1998). Inside "Pandora's box": Abused women's experiences with clinicians and health services. *Journal of General Internal Medicine*, *13*, 549–555.

Murdoch, M., Pryor, J. B., Polusny, M. A., & Gackstetter, G. D. (2007). Functioning and psychiatric symptoms among military men and women exposed to sexual stressors. *Military Medicine*, *172*, 718–725.

Pearlman, L. A., & Courtois, C. A. (2005). Clinical applications of the attachment framework: Relational treatment of complex trauma. *Journal of Traumatic Stress*, *18*, 449–459.

Rennison, C. M. (2002). *Rape and sexual assault: Reporting to police and medical attention. 1992–2000.* (NCJ Publication No. 194530), Washington, DC: Bureau of Justice Statistics.

Street, A. E., Gradus, J. L., Stafford, J., & Kelly, K. (2007). Gender differences in experiences of sexual harassment: Data from a male-dominated environment. *Journal of Consulting and Clinical Psychology*, *75*, 464–474.

Street, A. E., Kimerling, R., Bell, M. E., & Pavao, J. (2011). Sexual harassment and sexual assault during military service. In J. Ruzek, P. Schnurr, J. Vasterling, & M. Friedman (Eds.), *Posttraumatic stress reactions: Caring for the veterans of the global war on terror* (pp. 131–150). Washington, DC: American Psychological Association Books.

Street, A. E., Stafford, J., Mahan, C. M., & Hendricks, A. (2008). Sexual harassment and assault experienced by reservists during military service: Prevalence and health correlates. *Journal of Rehabilitation Research and Development*, *45*, 409–420.

Sugg, N. K., & Inui, T. (1992). Primary care physicians' response to domestic violence: Opening Pandora's box. *Journal of the American Medical Association*, *267*, 3157–3160.

Suris, A., & Lind, L. (2008). Military sexual trauma: A review of prevalence and associated health consequences in veterans. *Trauma, Violence & Abuse*, *9*(4), 250–269.

Suris, A. M., Lind, L., Kashner, T. M., & Borman, P. D. (2007). Mental health quality of life, and health functioning in women veterans: Differential outcomes associated with military and civilian sexual assault. *Journal of Interpersonal Violence*, *22*(2), 179–197.

Tjaden, P., & Thoennes, N. (2000). Prevalence and consequence of male-to-female and female-to-male intimate partner violence as measured by the National Violence Against Women Survey. *Violence Against Women*, *6*(2), 142–161.

Veterans Health Administration. (2005). *Military sexual trauma counseling* (VHA Directive No. 2005-015). Washington, DC: Department of Veterans Affairs.

Veterans Health Administration. (2008). *Uniform mental health services in VA medical centers and clinics* (VHA Handbook 1160.01). Washington, DC: Department of Veterans Affairs.

Zinzow, H. M., Grubaugh, A. L., Frueh, B. C., & Magruder, K. M. (2008). Sexual assault, mental health, and service use among male and female veterans seen in Veterans Affairs primary care clinics: A multi-site study. *Psychiatry Research*, *159*(1–2), 226–236.

Military Sexual Trauma in Men: A Review of Reported Rates

TIM HOYT, PhD, JENNIFER KLOSTERMAN RIELAGE, PhD, and LAUREN F. WILLIAMS, PhD

Behavioral Health Care Line, New Mexico Veterans Affairs Health Care System, Albuquerque, New Mexico, USA

Military sexual trauma (MST) has historically been associated with female service members, but it is also experienced by male service members. This article reviews reported prevalence and incidence rates of men's MST in 29 studies. Sources for these studies included the Department of Defense, the U.S. military service academies, and the Department of Veterans Affairs. There is significant variability in reported rates of men's MST. Averaging across studies covering the past 30 years, we found that MST is reported by approximately 0.09% of male service members each year, with a range of 0.02% to 6%. MST is reported by 1.1% of male service members over the course of their military careers, with a range of 0.03% to 12.4%. Determining prevalence and incidence rates for both men's and women's MST is fraught with limitations, including (a) cross-study variations in sample, method, definitions, and assessment and (b) barriers to reporting MST. Each of these limitations is reviewed with an eye toward identifying male-specific issues.

Tim Hoyt is now at the Department of Psychology, Madigan Army Medical Center, Ft. Lewis, Washington, USA.

The authors acknowledge and thank the anonymous reviewers of this article, as well as Kathleen Haaland and an anonymous veteran with military sexual trauma for their comments on previous versions of this article. This research was supported by the New Mexico Veterans Affairs Health Care System Research and Development program and a Department of Veterans Affairs Veterans Integrated Service Network New Investigator Grant awarded to the second author.

When the diagnosis of posttraumatic stress disorder (PTSD) was included in the *Diagnostic and Statistical Manual of Mental Disorders* (3rd ed.), gender-specific stressors were hypothesized to be associated with the disorder (see Herman, 1997). For men, exposure to combat could result in PTSD; for women, PTSD typically resulted from sexual trauma. Within this historical context, many practitioners may not recognize that men experience PTSD symptoms as the result of a rape or sexual assault. Research on military sexual trauma (MST) has identified significantly higher reported prevalence and incidence rates in women than in men (e.g., Kimerling, Gima, Smith, Street, & Frayne, 2007). Researchers and clinicians should take care not to assume that the lower reported MST prevalence rates in male veterans implies that men's MST is not a problem. The number of MST cases in men versus women identified in the Department of Veterans Affairs Health Care System (VA) is very similar (Turner & Frayne, 2004). In fiscal year 2003, VA universal screening identified 31,797 cases of men's MST and 29,418 cases of women's MST (Kimerling et al., 2007). In fiscal year 2005, universal screening identified 6,227 additional cases of men's MST and 6,469 cases of women's MST (Kimerling, Street, Gima, & Smith, 2008).

VA policy emphasizes the importance of MST treatment for both women and men and includes provisions for both male and female veterans to receive free services for MST, but specific guidelines for treatment are vague (Department of Veterans Affairs, 2008; Turner & Frayne, 2004). Indeed, there is no guideline for what MST services must be available, and men with MST generally have not received the same level of support as women (Leskela, Dieperink, & Kok, 2001).

Previous research on the MST indicates serious sequelae in both men and women (Kimerling et al., 2007; Magley, Waldo, Drasgow, & Fitzgerald, 1999). Sexual harassment of men in the military has shown a stronger association with emotional problems and decreases in work productivity than sexual harassment of women (Magley et al., 1999). In another study, men with MST were more likely than women with MST to be diagnosed with anxiety disorders other than PTSD, bipolar disorder, personality disorders, and psychosis (Kimerling et al., 2007). Psychological symptoms also appear to be more persistent and treatment resistant after MST in men than in women (O'Brien, Gaher, Pope, & Smiley, 2008).

The tendency to emphasize the treatment of women's MST over men's may be reflective of the acceptance of rape myths among providers (Kassing & Prieto, 2003; Shechory & Idisis, 2006). These rape myths include beliefs such as men are too strong to be overpowered, men are only raped in prison, and sexual trauma is worse for women than for men (Donnelly &

Kenyon, 1996; Groth & Burgess, 1980). Some clinicians also assume that MST only happens to men with childhood sexual trauma histories or personality disorders (Davies, 2002), or that men can only be raped by other men (Struckman-Johnson & Struckman-Johnson, 1992). These myths are similar to many rape myths that have been identified in women's sexual assault, but they may differ substantially in the recurrent themes involving the loss of masculinity often associated with men's sexual trauma (Groth & Burgess, 1980). It is possible that the lack of empirical work on men's MST is a result of these prevailing myths (Polusny & Murdoch, 2005).

This article reviews reported prevalence and incidence rates of men's MST and discusses barriers to the disclosure of men's MST that may affect reported rates. The methodology for this review was based on previous reviews of MST (e.g., Suris & Lind, 2008). Sources were identified through PsychLit, MEDLINE, OVID, the Defense Manpower Data Center, and the Department of Defense (DoD) Office of Sexual Assault Prevention and Response. The following key words were used in the search: *rape*, *sexual assault*, *military*, *harassment*, and *sexual trauma*. This search resulted in 210 relevant sources. Studies were excluded if they did not report data on sexual assault, did not provide data on male victims, focused on childhood sexual assault, or focused on qualitative descriptions. Exclusion resulted in a sample of 23 sources. References and citing articles for these sources provided six additional sources. The final sample consisted of 29 studies from the DoD, military service academies, and VA that reported prevalence or incidence rates of sexual assault against men during military service (see Tables 1 and 2).

The first decade of DoD research on MST in servicemen showed consistent reported rates less than 1% (Bastian, Lancaster, & Reyst, 1996; Culbertson, Rosenfeld, Booth-Kewley, & Magnusson, 1992; Culbertson, Rosenfeld, & Newell, 1993; Goyer & Eddleman, 1984; Martindale, 1990). During the 1990s, studies of men's MST showed greater variability, with reported rates ranging from 2% to 9% (Army Senior Review Panel on Sexual Harassment, 1997; Martin, Rosen, Durand, Stretch, & Knudson, 1998; Shipherd, Pineles, Gradus, & Resick, 2009). Since 2004, Public Laws 108-375 (Ronald W. Reagan National Defense Authorization Act for Fiscal Year 2005) and 109-364 (John Warner National Defense Authorization Act for Fiscal Year 2007) have required a yearly report to the U.S. Congress on sexual assault in the military and at the service academies, respectively. Although DoD reports for calendar years 2004–2006 did not provide a breakdown by victim sex, significant reported rate increases for formally reported men's sexual assault were identified by comparing 2007 and 2008 data with data from subsequent years ($z = 2.63$–8.81, $p < .01$; DoD, 2005, 2006a, 2007a, 2008, 2009b, 2010). Weighted sample surveys during this period show reported incidence rates between 0.9 and 2.0 (Lipari, Cook, Rock, & Matos, 2008; Lipari & Lancaster, 2003; Lipari, Lancaster, & Jones, 2005; Rock & Lipari, 2009).

TABLE 1 Reported Rates for 12-Month Incidence of Men's MST

Source	Group	Definition	*N* (men)	Cases	%	% Nonresponse	Other factors
Martindale (1990)	DoD	12-month incidence of rape or attempted rape "from someone where you work."	10, 752	38	0.4	40	Mailed survey to a stratified sample.
Culbertson et al. (1992)	Navy	Rape or attempted rape while on duty, or on base or ship in the past year.	2, 966	12[a]	0.4	40	Mailed survey to a stratified sample.
Culbertson et al. (1993)	Navy	Rape or attempted rape while on duty, or on base or ship while off duty in the past year.	2, 667[a]	13[a]	0.5	52	Mailed survey to a stratified sample.
Bastian et al. (1996)	DoD	12-month incidence of rape or attempted rape "from someone where you work" reported by men.	5, 913	12[a]	0.2	39	Mailed survey to a stratified sample. Decrease compared to Martindale (1990).
Army Senior Review Panel on Sexual Harassment (1997)	Army	"Someone having made attempts to have sex with you which resulted in you struggling; or having sex with you without your consent" in the past 12 months.	11, 816	708	6	40	Anonymous survey of companies at 59 posts; 14% of reported incidents occurred during IET.
Lipari & Lancaster (2003)	DoD	How often during the past 12 months have you been in situations involving military personnel or employees who had sex or attempted to have sex with you but was not successful, without your consent or against your will?	9, 980[a]	958[a]	1	68	Online survey with paper follow-up of stratified sample.
Lipari et al. (2005)	DoD	See Lipari & Lancaster (2003).	13, 686[a]	274[a]	2	64	Online survey with paper follow-up of stratified sample; reserve components.

(Continued)

TABLE 1 (Continued)

Source	Group	Definition	*N* (men)	Cases	%	% Nonresponse	Other factors
Cook et al. (2005)	Service academies	(In the past year) has someone done any of the following to you without your consent and against your will? 1) Touched, stroked, or fondled your private parts? 2) Physically attempted to have sexual intercourse with you, but was not successful? 3) Physically attempted to have oral or anal sex with you, but was not successful? 4) Had sexual intercourse with you? 5) Had oral sex with you?6) Had anal sex with you?	3, 287	86[a]	2.6	15	2004–2005 academic year. Anonymous survey to groups of cadets.
Lipari et al. (2006)	Service academies	(In the past year) have you experienced any of the following that were against your will or when you could not consent: 1) Sexually touched you or made you sexually touch them? 2) Attempted to make you have sexual intercourse, but was not successful? 3) Made you have sexual intercourse? 4) Made you perform or receive oral sex, anal sex, or penetration by a finger or object, or 5) Attempted to and was not successful?	3,969	60[a]	1.5	14	2005–2006 academic year. Anonymous paper survey to groups of cadets.
Cook & Lipari (2008)	Service academies	See Lipari et al. (2006).	2, 568	36	1.4	27	Anonymous paper survey.

Lipari et al. (2008)	DoD	See Lipari et al. (2006).	16, 433	296[a]	1.8	71	Online survey with paper follow-up to a stratified sample.
DoD (2008)	DoD	Reports to victim advocate of rape, attempted rape, sodomy, or indecent assault during FY2007 (male SM victim).	1, 170, 264[b]	125	0.017	NR	Restricted and unrestricted reports to victim advocates. SM perpetrator.
DoD (2009a)	DoD	Reports to victim advocate of rape, attempted rape, sodomy, or indecent assault during FY2008 (male SM victim).	1, 190, 468[b]	173	0.015	NR	Restricted and unrestricted reports to victim advocates. SM perpetrator.
Shipherd et al. (2009)	Marines	Sexual coercion, attempted or completed rape in the past 6 months.	323	29	9.0	58	Mailed follow-up survey of 1997 Marine cohort.
Rock & Lipari (2009)	DoD	See Lipari et al. (2006).	11, 367[a]	102[a]	0.9	66	Online survey with paper follow-up of stratified sample; reserve components.
DoD (2010)	DoD	Reports to victim advocate of rape, attempted rape, sodomy, or indecent assault during FY2009.	1, 204, 060[b]	384	0.032	NR	Restricted and unrestricted reports to victim advocates.
Total			3, 660, 519	3, 306	0.090	45	Weighted mean percentages.

Notes. MST = military sexual trauma; DoD = Department of Defense; IET = Initial Entry Training (e.g., Basic Combat Training or Advanced Individual Training); FY = fiscal year; SM = service member; NR = not reported.

[a]Estimate based on weighting and sample stratification. [b]Estimated population for calendar/academic year based on Defense Manpower Data Center (2010).

TABLE 2 Rates for Prevalence of Men's Sexual Assault During Military Service

Source	Group	Definition	*N* (men)	Cases	%	% Nonresponse	Other factors
Goyer & Eddleman (1984)	Navy	Male–male rape by another SM.	2,890	7	0.4	NR	Review of outpatient medical records. Limited to men specifically seeking medical services related to assault.
Army Senior Review Panel on Sexual Harassment (1997)	Army	"Someone having made attempts to have sex with you which resulted in you struggling; or having sex with you without your consent" since enlisting in the Army.	4,228	85	2	NR	Anonymous survey at 14 Initial Entry Training facilities.
Martin et al. (1998)	Army	Rape, attempted rape, or attempted unwanted and forced sexual contact after entering the military.	555	18	3.2	NR	Participants were provided by units after requests for involvement in large-scale screening on six Army posts.
Smith et al. (1999)	VA	Lifetime sexual assault, including "prior to combat experience."	129	16	12.4	NR	Interview with combat veterans referred for PTSD evaluation.
Department of the Air Force (2003)	Air Force Academy	Investigated allegation of rape, attempted rape, sodomy, or indecent assault (male cadet victim).	10,080[a]	3	0.029	NR	Cases reported between 1993 and 2002 at the Air Force Academy.
Department of the Air Force (2003)	Air Force Academy	"Have you ever been sexually assaulted since you arrived at the U.S. Air Force Academy?"	3,547	61	1.7	58.6	Review of data from the Social Climate Survey at the Air Force Academy in survey years 1996, 1997, 1998, 2000, and 2002. Rates of nonresponse ranged from 21% to 92%.

Murdoch et al. (2004)	VA	Someone attempted or forced the victim to have sex against his will during military service.	1,654	70	4.2	32.1	Mailed survey to veterans seeking disability benefits.
Naval Inspector General (2004)	Navy	"Since you have joined the Navy, has anyone done any of the following actions without your consent and against your will: touched privates, attempted (oral/anal) sex, had (oral/anal) sex?"	27,852	1,181	4.0	10	Internet-based study sent to 10% of the active duty Navy.
OIG (2005)	Service academies	Since becoming a cadet/midshipman, has someone done any of the following to you without your consent and against your will? Touched, stroked, or fondled your private parts, physically attempted to have sexual (anal/oral) intercourse with you but was not successful, had sexual (oral/anal) intercourse with you.	3,107	54	1.7	3	Random sample of approximately one third of cadets/midshipmen between 1999 and 2004.
Kang et al. (2005)	VA	"Suffered forced sexual relations or a sexual assault" while in the Persian Gulf.	9,310	19[a]	0.2	23.7	Mailed initial survey, with follow-up phone interview.
Hough & DeGirolamo (2007)	VA	See Kimerling et al. (2007)	297	5	1.7	10.1	Screened for MST during VA intake interview for spinal injury program.

(*Continued*)

TABLE 2 (Continued)

Source	Group	Definition	*N* (men)	Cases	%	% Nonresponse	Other factors
Kimerling et al. (2007)	VA	"While you were in the military: Did you receive uninvited and unwanted sexual attention, such as touching, cornering, pressure for sexual favors, or verbal remarks?; or Did someone ever use force or threat of force to have sexual contact with you against your will?"	2, 900, 106	31, 797	1.1	29.3	All responses to universal VA screening for PTSD during FY2003.
Street et al. (2008)	NG/R	At least one experience of coerced genital fondling, attempted rape, or completed rape during service in Reserve components.	1, 628	26[a]	1.6	15.8	Phone interview.
Kimerling et al. (2008)	VA	See Kimerling et al. (2007).	540, 381	6, 227	1.2	NR	All valid responses to the 2005 universal VA MST screening.13.3% of the VA census was not included in this universal screen.
Haskell et al. (2010)	VA	See Kimerling et al. (2007).	1, 032	6	0.6	NR	Connecticut sample from VA database.
Total			3, 506, 796	39, 575	1.1	22.8	Weighted mean percentages.

Notes. SM = service member; NR = not reported; VA = Veterans Affairs; PTSD = posttraumatic stress disorder; OIG = Office of the Inspector General of the Department of Defense; MST = military sexual trauma; FY = fiscal year; NG/R = National Guard and Reserve.

[a]Estimate based on weighting and sample stratification. [b]Estimated population for calendar/academic year based on Defense Manpower Data Center (2010).

Yearly social climate surveys from the military service academies suggest a stable reported rate between 1% and 2% over the past decade (Cook, Jones, Lipari, & Lancaster, 2005; Cook & Lipari, 2008; DoD, 2007b; Department of the Air Force, 2003; Lipari et al., 2006; Office of the Inspector General of the Department of Defense [OIG], 2005). Universal screening for MST among men in the VA shows similar reported rates of 1.1% to 1.2% (Kimerling et al., 2007, 2008). Smaller samples from the VA show greater variability, with reported rates ranging from 0.2% to 12%, using the VA screening question and other assessment instruments (Haskell et al., 2010; Hough & DeGirolamo, 2007; Kang, Dalager, Mahan, & Ishii, 2005; Murdoch Polusny, Hodges, & O'Brien, 2004; Smith, Frueh, Sawchuk, & Johnson, 1999; Street, Stafford, Mahan, & Hendricks, 2008).

EXAMINING REPORTED RATES OF MEN'S MST

In summary, reported rates of men's MST across studies in the DoD, military service academies, and VA range from 0.02% to 12%, with a weighted average of 0.09% for 12-month incidence and 1.1% for lifetime prevalence. Studies on formally investigated sexual assault show a significantly lower reported rate (0.6%) than anonymous surveys (2.8%; $z = 111.09$, $p < .001$). DoD studies (0.1%) estimate reported rates significantly lower than reported rates identified in VA studies (1.1%; $z = 169.12$, $p < .001$). However, this difference does not take sample bias into account, as not every veteran enrolls at VA facilities (Congressional Budget Office, 2005). Variability in reported rates of MST also appears to decrease when the same item or measure is utilized (e.g., Kimerling et al., 2007, 2008) but increase when studies that used differing assessment instruments or methodology are compared.

Rates of nonresponse ranged from 3% to 92%, depending on the context of the survey. Estimates suggest that 66% of men's sexual assault incidents are not formally reported (Naval Inspector General, 2004). Overlapping data from surveys and crime reports suggest that only 10% of sexual assaults on men at the service academies are reported (Cook & Lipari, 2008; DoD, 2009a). A portion of nonrespondents may be avoiding thinking or talking about an assault or may prefer not to disclose the event. A number of other factors may influence rates of nonresponse, including the length of questionnaires, the substantial number of surveys conducted by the military, and the perception that surveys of this kind have no impact on military policy (Newell, Rosenfeld, Harris, & Hindelang, 2004). The lowest nonresponse rates were seen in service academy studies with mandatory participation (OIG, 2005). However, mandatory completion requirements also may contribute to invalid data, such as cadet men reporting "assault by vaginal penetration" (Department of the Air Force, 2003, Footnote 220). Universal screening in the VA system provides accountability to ensure that each veteran has the opportunity to report whether he has experienced MST (Kimerling et al., 2007, 2008). Nonetheless, universal screening does not ensure that women or men will report accurately. Veterans also may decline to answer questions assessing MST, and procedures for universal screening vary significantly (Street, Kelly, & Kimerling, 2006). Nonetheless, universal screening appears to be most effective at both identifying consistent rates of MST as well as connecting victims of MST to clinical services. It is possible that a similar universal screening procedure could be implemented as part of the yearly periodic health assessment for active duty service members (see DoD, 2006b). This addition may increase the DoD's ability to identify accurate rates of MST and connect victims to clinical services.

In addition to variations in screening methods, there has been inconsistency in the definition and assessment of MST (see Tables 1 and 2). Some reports excluded sexual assault data (e.g., Thomas, Newell, & Eliassen, 1995), whereas others emphasized associated behaviors (e.g., stalking; Lipari et al., 2006). As another illustration, current DoD interpretation of annual reporting requirements under Public Law 109-364 indicates that detailed surveys and focus groups will be conducted only biannually (DoD, 2009a). When detailed surveys were not conducted, reports emphasized compliance with DoD policy rather than sexual assault incidence (DoD, 2007b, 2009a). There also has been significant variation in items assessing men's MST. In some cases, the inclusion of several qualitative categories (e.g., unwanted contact, coerced intercourse) may better identify disparate incidents (Cook & Lipari, 2008). However, research on men's MST tends to group these qualitatively different occurrences into single items because of relatively low frequency (OIG, 2005). For example, some surveys used a single item measure of both sexual harassment and abuse (Fontana, Litz, & Rosenheck, 2000). Other studies excluded in-depth data on men's MST because of low reported rates (e.g., Culbertson et al., 1993). In the future, reporting frequency data on specific items may alleviate measurement inconsistency.

BARRIERS TO DISCLOSURE

Several barriers may discourage the reporting of MST for both men and women. Niebuhr (1997) suggested that the need for cohesion in military units may discourage people from reporting MST. Men who disclose MST or accuse their attackers during their military service can face ridicule, accusations that they are gay, or charges of fraternization or other associated behaviors (e.g., underage drinking) under the Uniform Code of Military Justice (Helle, 2004; Nelson, 2002). In contrast, criminal action against perpetrators can be delayed by investigation processes, sending messages that the victim rather than the perpetrator is being punished or that perpetrators are unlikely to be punished (Cook & Lipari, 2008; Nuwer, 2004). Withdrawn reports can also give victims the perception that they will not be believed (Cook & Lipari, 2008).

The unique culture in the military promotes discipline, loyalty, and collectivism—values that may discourage service members from reporting sexual assault committed by fellow service members (Department of the Air Force, 2003). When sexual assault is reported, victims may feel ostracized or may be openly attacked in acts of retaliation by perpetrators, peers, and the chain of command. In some cases, male victims of MST report being threatened with death if they report the incident (Nuwer, 2004). Access to weapons in the military, a prominent feature in many accounts of men's MST, adds lethal potential to fears of retribution (Hunter, 2007). In other situations, violations of the "code of silence" may be perceived when hazing rituals are disclosed because an initiate experienced MST (Nuwer, 2004). Commonly cited reasons for not reporting incidents for both men and women include embarrassment, fear of reprisal through duty evaluations, a belief that the incident was "not important enough" to report, and fear that nothing will be done (Bastian et al., 1996). Some victims of MST who reported the incident describe violations of privacy when subsequent commanders and fellow service members learned details of the assault years later through service records (Nelson, 2002).

Pressure for men to be "stoic warriors" by denying pain and suppressing emotions may further prevent victims from seeking help (Sherman, 2005). A significant part of training for combat is learning emotional control. The emotional upheaval associated with MST may cause service members to feel that they are not in control of their emotions and in turn that they are not "worthy" to serve in the military (Turner & Frayne, 2004). Well-meaning commanders may reassign victims of MST to other tasks, effectively removing them from their military duties (Nelson, 2002). This may create pressure for service members to "soldier on" or deny health problems to avoid reassignment (Mullins, 2005). Similarly, male veterans with MST may feel that the "manhood" earned through military service has been stolen from them (Hopper, 2006). Because of this, male veterans who have experienced MST may be more likely to seek treatment for health problems rather than psychological symptoms (Kimerling et al., 2007). This focus on physical complaints may result from perceptions that disclosing MST threatens masculinity by sharing feelings or seeking help (Hopper, 2006). These feelings of machismo also can be prominent in Hispanic veterans (Canive, Castillo, & Tuason, 2001). Men who have been sexually assaulted also may experience sexual identity confusion, potentially leading to concerns regarding their military careers under prior "Don't Ask, Don't Tell" policies (Moradi & Miller, 2010). Because constructs such as stoicism and hypermasculinity appear related to rates of MST disclosure, active challenging of these values within military culture and veterans' treatment facilities may be warranted. Instead, military values such as bravery, loyalty, and discipline can be promoted.

These values may encourage disclosure and treatment seeking (Hopper, 2006).

Examining patterns of reporting over the past 30 years suggests that reported rates of MST are increasing. It has been suggested that this trend does not reflect an increase in the occurrence of MST (DoD, 2009b, 2010). Rather, it is possible that improved reporting practices make it possible for men to report sexual assaults with fewer stigmas. Policy changes by the DoD during the past decade may have played a role in increased reporting. For example, the DoD published specific guidelines establishing sexual assault response coordinator positions to facilitate the reporting of sexual assault (DoD, 2006c). These guidelines also established the infrastructure for round-the-clock responses by victim advocates down to the unit level.

In order to encourage the disclosure of MST, screening should become routine in clinical practice (Polusny & Murdoch, 2005). This entails asking veterans regularly whether they have experienced MST, even if the initial assessment was negative. Clinicians should communicate to veterans during routine screenings that the victim is not the only one who has experienced MST, that he is not responsible for what happened, and that symptoms of PTSD following MST are common (Valente & Wight, 2007). Further keys to facilitating disclosure of MST include being compassionate, being sensitive, being nonjudgmental, and maintaining privacy and confidentiality (Lineberry, Bostwick, Ramaswamy, & Rundell, 2006).

SUMMARY

MST remains a prevalent issue for both men and women, and there appear to be important gender differences in both reported rates of MST and associated sequelae. Research on men's MST over the past 30 years has been limited by significant variations in methodology and barriers to disclosure. Both researchers and clinicians identifying and treating cases involving men's MST should be aware of these factors and work to overcome barriers associated with the accurate identification of sexual trauma in male service members. We hope that this summary of the research on men's MST can raise awareness of this issue and ultimately improve clinical services for these men.

REFERENCES

Army Senior Review Panel on Sexual Harassment. (1997). *The Secretary of the Army's senior review panel report on sexual harassment*. Washington, DC: Department of the Army.

Bastian, L., Lancaster, A., & Reyst, H. (1996). *Department of Defense 1995 sexual harassment survey*. Arlington, VA: Defense Manpower Data Center.

Canive, J., Castillo, D., & Tuason, V. (2001). The Hispanic veteran. In W. Tseng & J. Streltzer (Eds.), *Culture and psychotherapy: A guide to clinical practice* (pp. 157–172). Washington, DC: American Psychiatric Press.

Congressional Budget Office. (2005). *The potential cost of meeting demand for veterans' health care*. Washington, DC: Author.

Cook, P., Jones, A., Lipari, R., & Lancaster, A. (2005). *Service academy 2005 sexual harassment and assault survey*. Arlington, VA: Defense Manpower Data Center.

Cook, P., & Lipari, R. (2008). *2008 service academy gender relations survey*. Arlington, VA: Defense Manpower Data Center.

Culbertson, A., Rosenfeld, P., Booth-Kewley, S., & Magnusson, P. (1992). *Assessment of sexual harassment in the Navy: Results of the 1989 Navy-wide survey*. San Diego, CA: Navy Personnel Research and Development Center.

Culbertson, A., Rosenfeld, P., & Newell, C. (1993). *Sexual harassment in the active-duty Navy: Findings from the 1991 Navy-wide survey*. San Diego, CA: Navy Personnel Research and Development Center.

Davies, M. (2002). Male sexual assault victims: A selective review of the literature and implications for support services. *Aggression and Violent Behavior, 7*, 203–214.

Defense Manpower Data Center. (2010). *DoD personnel and procurement statistics*. Retrieved from http://siadapp.dmdc.osd.mil

Department of Defense. (2005). *Calendar year 2004 report: Sexual offenses involving members of the armed forces*. Washington, DC: Author.

Department of Defense. (2006a). *Calendar year 2005 report: Sexual offenses involving members of the armed forces*. Washington, DC: Author.

Department of Defense. (2006b). *Health Affairs Policy 06-006: Periodic health assessment policy for active duty and selected reserve members*. Washington, DC: Author.

Department of Defense. (2006c). *Sexual assault prevention and response program procedures* (DoD Instruction No. 6495.02). Washington, DC: Author.

Department of Defense. (2007a). *Annual report on military services sexual assault for calendar year 2006*. Washington, DC: Author.

Department of Defense. (2007b). *Report on sexual harassment and violence at the U.S. military service academies: Academic program year 2006-2007*. Washington, DC: Author.

Department of Defense. (2008). *FY07 report on sexual assault in the military*. Washington, DC: Author.

Department of Defense. (2009a). *Annual report on sexual harassment and violence at the U.S. military service academies: Academic program year 2008-2009*. Washington, DC: Author.

Department of Defense. (2009b). *FY08 report on sexual assault in the military*. Washington, DC: Author.

Department of Defense. (2010). *Fiscal year 2009 annual report on sexual assault in the military*. Washington, DC: Author.

Department of the Air Force. (2003). *The report of the working group concerning the deterrence of and response to incidents of sexual assault at the U.S. Air Force Academy*. Washington, DC: Author.

Department of Veterans Affairs. (2008). *Uniform mental health services in VA medical centers and clinics* (VHA Handbook No. 1160.01). Washington, DC: Author.

Donnelly, D., & Kenyon, S. (1996). "Honey, we don't do men": Gender stereotypes and the provision of services to sexually assaulted males. *Journal of Interpersonal Violence, 11*, 441–448.

Fontana, A., Litz, B., & Rosenheck, R. (2000). Impact of combat and sexual harassment on the severity of posttraumatic stress disorder among men and women peacekeepers in Somalia. *Journal of Nervous and Mental Disease, 188,* 163–169.

Goyer, P., & Eddleman, H. (1984). Same-sex rape of nonincarcerated men. *American Journal of Psychiatry, 141*, 576–579.

Groth, A., & Burgess, A. (1980). Male rape: Offenders and victims. *American Journal of Psychiatry, 137*, 806–810.

Haskell, S., Gordon, K., Mattocks, K., Duggal, M., Erdos, J., Justice, A., & Brandt, C. (2010). Gender differences in rates of depression, PTSD, pain, obesity, and military sexual trauma among Connecticut war veterans of Iraq and Afghanistan. *Journal of Women's Health, 19*, 267–271.

Helle, G. (2004). *The enemy within: One Vietnam veteran helps others cope with PTSD*. Bloomington, IN: Authorhouse.

Herman, J. (1997). *Trauma and recovery*. New York, NY: Basic Books.

Hopper, J. (2006, June). *Male victims: Special issues*. Paper presented at the Sexual Assault Response Coordinator conference, St. Louis, MO.

Hough, S., & DeGirolamo, S. (2007). The experience of military sexual trauma and rehabilitation for individuals with spinal cord injury/dysfunction. *Sexuality and Disability, 25*, 65–72.

Hunter, M. (2007). *Honor betrayed: Sexual abuse in America's military*. Fort Lee, NJ: Barricade Books.

John Warner National Defense Authorization Act for Fiscal Year 2007, Pub. L. No. 109-364, 120 Stat. 2083 (2006).

Kang, H., Dalager, N., Mahan, C., & Ishii, E. (2005). The role of sexual assault on the risk of PTSD among Gulf War veterans. *Annals of Epidemiology, 15*, 191–195.

Kassing, L., & Prieto, L. (2003). The rape myth and blame-based beliefs of counselors-in-training toward male victims of rape. *Journal of Counseling & Development, 81*, 455–461.

Kimerling, R., Gima, K., Smith, M., Street, A., & Frayne, S. (2007). The Veterans Health Administration and military sexual trauma. *American Journal of Public Health, 97*, 2160–2166.

Kimerling, R., Street, A., Gima, K., & Smith, M. (2008). Evaluation of universal screening for military-related sexual trauma. *Psychiatric Services, 59*, 635–640.

Leskela, J., Dieperink, M., & Kok, C. (2001). Group treatment with sexually assaulted male veterans: A year in review. *Group, 25*, 303–319.

Lineberry, T., Bostwick, J., Ramaswamy, S., & Rundell, J. (2006). Military sexual trauma: How to identify and treat a unique form of PTSD. *Current Psychiatry, 5*, 53–54.

Lipari, R., Cook, P., Rock, L., & Matos, K. (2008). *2006 gender relations survey of active duty members*. Arlington, VA: Defense Manpower Data Center.

Lipari, R., & Lancaster, A. (2003). *Armed forces 2002 sexual harassment survey*. Arlington, VA: Defense Manpower Data Center.

Lipari, R., Lancaster, A., & Jones, A. (2005). *2004 sexual harassment survey of reserve component members*. Arlington, VA: Defense Manpower Data Center.

Lipari, R., Wessels, K., Cook, P., Jones, A., Pennington, J., & Kidwell, E. (2006). *Service academy 2006 gender relations survey*. Arlington, VA: Defense Manpower Data Center.

Magley, V., Waldo, C., Drasgow, F., & Fitzgerald, L. (1999). The impact of sexual harassment on military personnel: Is it the same for men and women? *Military Psychology, 11*, 283–302.

Martin, L., Rosen, L., Durand, D., Stretch, R., & Knudson, K. (1998). Prevalence and timing of sexual assaults in a sample of male and female U.S. Army soldiers. *Military Medicine, 163*, 213–216.

Martindale, M. (1990). *Sexual harassment in the military: 1988*. Arlington, VA: Defense Manpower Data Center.

Moradi, B., & Miller, L. (2010). Attitudes of Iraq and Afghanistan War veterans toward gay and lesbian service members. *Armed Forces and Society, 36*, 397–419.

Mullins, C. (2005). Understanding sexual assault in the United States military culture. *Connections, 7*, 8–11.

Murdoch, M., Polusny, M., Hodges, J., & O'Brien, N. (2004). Prevalence of in-service and post-service sexual assault among combat and noncombat veterans applying for Department of Veterans Affairs posttraumatic stress disorder disability benefits. *Military Medicine, 169*, 392–395.

Naval Inspector General. (2004). *NAVINSGEN sexual assault study*. Washington, DC: Department of the Navy.

Nelson, T. (2002). *For love of country: Confronting rape and sexual harassment in the U.S. military*. New York, NY: Haworth Press.

Newell, C., Rosenfeld, P., Harris, R., & Hindelang, R. (2004). Reasons for non-response on U.S. Navy surveys: A closer look. *Military Psychology, 16*, 265–276.

Niebuhr, R. (1997). Sexual harassment in the military. In W. O'Donohue (Ed.), *Sexual harassment: Theory, research, and treatment* (pp. 250–262). Needham Heights, MA: Allyn & Bacon.

Nuwer, H. (2004). Military hazing. In H. Nuwer (Ed.), *The hazing reader* (pp. 141–146). Bloomington: Indiana University Press.

O'Brien, C., Gaher, R., Pope, C., & Smiley, P. (2008). Difficulty identifying feelings predicts persistence of trauma symptoms in a sample of veterans who experienced military sexual trauma. *Journal of Nervous and Mental Disease, 196*, 252–255.

Office of the Inspector General of the Department of Defense. (2005). *Report on the service academy sexual assault and leadership survey*. Arlington, VA: Author.

Polusny, M., & Murdoch, M. (2005). Sexual assault among male veterans. *Psychiatric Times, 22*, 34–37.

Rock, L., & Lipari, R. (2009). *2008 gender relations survey of reserve component members*. Arlington, VA: Defense Manpower Data Center.

Ronald W. Reagan National Defense Authorization Act for Fiscal Year 2005, Pub. L. No. 108-375, 118 Stat. 1181 (2004).

Shechory, M., & Idisis, Y. (2006). Rape myths and social distance toward sex offenders and victims among therapists and students. *Sex Roles, 54*, 651–658.

Sherman, N. (2005). *Stoic warriors: The ancient philosophy behind the military mind*. New York, NY: Oxford University Press.

Shipherd, J., Pineles, S., Gradus, J., & Resick, P. (2009). Sexual harassment in the Marines, posttraumatic stress symptoms, and perceived health: Evidence for sex differences. *Journal of Traumatic Stress*, *22*, 3–10.

Smith, D., Frueh, B., Sawchuk, C., & Johnson, M. (1999). Relationship between symptom over-reporting and pre- and post-combat trauma history in veterans evaluated for PTSD. *Depression and Anxiety*, *10*, 119–124.

Street, A., Kelly, K., & Kimerling, R. (2006). *National survey of military sexual trauma practice summary report*. Washington, DC: Department of Veterans Affairs.

Street, A., Stafford, J., Mahan, C., & Hendricks, A. (2008). Sexual harassment and assault experienced by reservists during military service: Prevalence and health correlates. *Journal of Rehabilitation Research and Development*, *45*, 409–419.

Struckman-Johnson, C., & Struckman-Johnson, D. (1992). Acceptance of male rape myths among college men and women. *Sex Roles*, *27*, 85–100.

Suris, A., & Lind, L. (2008). Military sexual trauma: A review of prevalence and associated health consequences in veterans. *Trauma, Violence, & Abuse*, *9*, 250–269.

Thomas, P., Newell, C., & Eliassen, D. (1995). *Sexual harassment of Navy personnel: Results of a 1993 survey*. San Diego, CA: Navy Personnel Research and Development Center.

Turner, C., & Frayne, S. (2004). *Military sexual trauma: Veterans health initiative independent study course*. Birmingham, AL: Department of Veterans Affairs.

Valente, S., & Wight, C. (2007). Military sexual trauma: Violence and sexual abuse. *Military Medicine*, *172*, 259–265.

Posttraumatic Sequelae Associated with Military Sexual Trauma in Female Veterans Enrolled in VA Outpatient Mental Health Clinics

JANE A. LUTEREK, PhD

Mental Health Service, VA Puget Sound Health Care System, Seattle, Washington; and Department of Psychiatry and Behavioral Sciences, University of Washington, Seattle, Washington, USA

JOYCE N. BITTINGER, MS

Department of Psychology, University of Washington, Seattle, Washington, USA

TRACY L. SIMPSON, PhD

Mental Health Service, VA Puget Sound Health Care System, Seattle, Washington; and Department of Psychiatry and Behavioral Sciences, University of Washington, Seattle, Washington, USA

The purpose of this study was to explore the relationship between military sexual assault (MSA) and posttraumatic stress disorder (PTSD) and other symptoms associated with trauma, referred to as disorders of extreme stress not otherwise specified (DESNOS) or complex PTSD within a Veterans Affairs (VA) Medical Center outpatient mental health treatment–seeking sample. The present results focus on female Veterans only because of the low rates of endorsement of MSA among male Veterans resulting in a sample too small to use in analyses. Compared with those who did not endorse MSA, those who did reported greater frequency of other potentially traumatic events; PTSD symptoms; and symptoms

The authors wish to thank the following individuals for conducting study interviews: Mary Jean Mariano, PhD; Lynne Hearle; Scott Michael, PhD; Victoria McKeever, PhD; and Jennifer Reilage, PhD.

This material is based upon work supported by a pilot grant from the Epidemiologic Research and Information Center, VA Puget Sound Health Care System, Office of Research and Development Cooperative Studies Program, Department of Veterans Affairs.

characteristic of DESNOS, such as difficulties with interpersonal relationships, emotion regulation, dissociation, somatization, and self-perception. When childhood and other adulthood interpersonal trauma were both taken into account, MSA continued to contribute unique variance in predicting PTSD and DESNOS symptoms. VA patients reporting MSA may represent notably heterogeneous groups that include more complex posttraumatic reactions. Treatment interventions focused on complex PTSD may be warranted for a subset of female veterans who endorse MSA.

The assessment and treatment of military sexual trauma (MST) has been a growing concern across the Veterans Health Administration and has received increased research attention over the past decade. Nationwide Veterans Health Administration policy requires documentation of MST screening and the provision of treatment services for conditions associated with MST. Consistent with the literature examining exposure to civilian adult sexual assault, MST has been associated with detrimental psychiatric symptoms, most notably increased rates of posttraumatic stress disorder (PTSD), depression, and alcohol abuse (see Surís & Lind, 2008, for a review). Women Veterans who endorse MST are more likely than their female counterparts with no history of MST to endorse symptoms of depression and alcohol abuse (Hankin et al., 1999; Surís, Lind, Kashner, & Borman, 2007) as well as PTSD (Himmelfarb, Yaeger, & Mintz, 2006; Surís et al., 2007; Surís, Lind, Kashner, Borman, & Petty, 2004; Wolfe et al., 1998; Yaeger, Himmelfarb, Cammack, & Mitz, 2006). Evidence suggests that female Veterans who experience MST are also at increased risk for developing PTSD relative to those who experience adult civilian sexual assault (Himmelfarb et al., 2006; Surís et al., 2004, 2007) and childhood sexual abuse (Surís et al., 2004). This same pattern is seen when other types of military trauma are examined, such that MST is associated with a greater risk of developing PTSD than are other types of duty-related stress (Fontana & Rosenheck, 1998; Wolfe et al., 1998; Yeager et al., 2006). Beyond psychiatric symptoms, MST has also been associated with significantly poorer physical health, life satisfaction with family relations, daily activities, and satisfaction with health than civilian sexual trauma (Surís et al., 2007). Taken together, these data suggest that the experience of MST may lead to particularly difficult posttraumatic sequelae.

Within a broader context, MST has also been associated with a lifetime history of interpersonal trauma, including childhood sexual abuse and sexual assault prior and subsequent to military service (Sadler, Booth, Mengeling, &

Doebbeling, 2004). Veterans have evidenced especially high rates of pre-military (Engel et al., 1993; King, King, Foy, & Gudanowski, 1996; King, King, Foy, Keane, & Fairbank, 1999), military (Fontana & Rosenheck, 1998; Fontana, Schwartz, & Rosenheck, 1997; Himmelfarb et al., 2006; Valente & Wright, 2007), and post-military (Murdoch, Polusny, Hodges, & O'Brien, 2004) interpersonal trauma exposure, much of which has been chronic in nature. While repeated trauma exposure has been related to an increased risk of developing PTSD (e.g., King et al., 1996, 1999), repeated, chronic, interpersonal trauma may also lead to adaptations associated with complex posttraumatic difficulties termed *disorders of extreme stress not otherwise specified* (DESNOS; Herman, 1992a; Roth, Newman, Pelcovitz, van der Kolk, & Mandel, 1997; van der Kolk, Roth, Pelcovitz, Sunday, & Spinazzola, 2005).

DESNOS is characterized by difficulties in affective, cognitive, biological, and relational domains following exposure to trauma (Pelcovitz et al., 1997), and symptoms have been found to be more prevalent in those with a history of early onset and longer lasting interpersonal trauma (van der Kolk et al., 2005). Specifically, DESNOS symptoms involve persistent difficulties in the following domains: (a) affect and impulse regulation (e.g., excessive risk taking), (b) somatization, (c) attention or consciousness (i.e., dissociation), (d) self-perception (i.e., viewing the self as damaged), (e) interpersonal relationships (e.g., impaired boundaries), and (f) sustaining beliefs (e.g., hopelessness). DESNOS symptoms have been associated with single-incident interpersonal trauma, and with more severe interpersonal trauma in a dose-respondent manner, and they have been shown to be independent from other trauma sequelae, including PTSD, affective disorders, and other anxiety disorders (Ford, Stockton, Kaltman, & Green, 2006). Previous research with male combat Veterans found that DESNOS was associated with childhood interpersonal trauma (Ford, 1999). Given previous evidence of increased posttraumatic sequelae associated with MST compared to other interpersonal traumas, and given the previously established relationship between interpersonal trauma and DESNOS, examining DESNOS symptomatology among these Veterans has the potential to characterize clinically meaningful subgroups of MST survivors. Such information may provide an evidence base for investigations of promising treatment approaches (e.g., dialectical behavior therapy; Wagner & Linehan, 2006; see also Courtois & Ford, 2009) that address emotion dysregulation and interpersonal problems typically attendant with DESNOS.

The purpose of the present study was to enhance our understanding of the clinical picture of those who present for outpatient mental health treatment at a Veterans Affairs (VA) Medical Center and who endorse MST. Although the Department of Veterans Affairs definition of MST includes severe or threatening forms of sexual harassment as well as sexual assault experienced during military service, we chose to focus on military sexual assault (MSA) as the trauma exposure measure used in this study did not provide contextual information on sexual harassment, such that neither its severity nor whether it was threatening in nature could be determined. At a basic level, we sought to replicate previous research on the relationship between MSA and exposure to potentially traumatic events, PTSD, and depression symptoms within an outpatient mental health treatment–seeking sample. Extending previous research, we sought to explore the potential relationship between MSA and DESNOS symptoms within this sample. Specifically, we hypothesized that MSA would be related to increased trauma exposure, PTSD, depression, and DESNOS symptoms and that MSA would be partially related to these measures of posttraumatic distress when childhood and other adulthood interpersonal trauma was controlled. In addition, given that typical samples endorse high rates of exposure to potentially traumatic events, we assessed patients' perceptions regarding whether MSA was their most distressing potentially traumatic experience, hypothesizing that those who endorse MSA as currently most distressing may struggle with greater posttraumatic sequelae.

METHOD

Participants

The study sample ($N = 208$) consisted of 104 female and 104 male Veterans recruited from the VA Puget Sound Health Care System (VAPSHCS) outpatient general mental health clinic (50%) and specialized mental health clinic for PTSD (50%). Participants engaged in addictions treatment or the outpatient clinic serving Veterans with severe chronic mental illness (e.g., schizophrenia, schizoaffective disorder) were not recruited for this study. An initial sample of 977 Veterans (500 males, 477 females) was identified from the VA Consumer Health Information Performance Sets VISN 20 regional data warehouse based on initial screening criteria. Male Veterans were randomly selected from the pool of those eligible, and all eligible female Veterans were selected. Participant inclusion criteria were as follows: (a) VAPSHCS enrollment for at least 12 months, (b) at least two mental health visits in the past year, and (c) being actively followed in the general mental health or PTSD clinic at the time of the assessment. Prior to the study, the primary mental health provider for each Veteran was contacted to determine whether the Veteran was sufficiently clinically stable to participate in the study. Clinicians were asked to use the following criteria to determine stability: patient is capable of providing informed consent, not currently receiving psychiatric inpatient care, not currently actively suicidal or homicidal, and does not currently have a flag indicating dangerousness in his or her VA medical record.

Of the initially identified sample ($n = 977$), 35% ($n = 338$) were never contacted, as recruitment efforts ended when the target sample size was achieved. Of the remaining 639,23% ($n = 147$) were considered ineligible by their primary mental health provider, 42% ($n = 269$) declined to participate in the study, and less than 2% ($n = 11$) did not attend the scheduled assessment. Of the 492 who were contacted and who were eligible, 214 (43%) completed the interview. Using the available demographics from the data warehouse (i.e., age, gender, race, and marital status), we found no significant differences between the study sample and those in the initial sample or who declined participation. We excluded 3 transgender individuals (1 of whom endorsed MSA) from the analyses because of the small number and 3 participants because of missing data on MSA history.

Procedure

Participants were contacted and scheduled for a single in-person session held at the VA facility. Participants completed self-report questionnaires and an interview during the study session. Interviews were conducted by a licensed psychologist or master's-level counselor. Interviewers underwent training by conducting mock interviews that were checked for fidelity. In addition, each interviewer's first two interviews were audiotaped and independently rated. Discrepancies between ratings were discussed with the interviewers so as to provide corrective information. The provider who did the vast majority of the interviews was also engaged in ongoing supervision in an effort to avoid bias and drift. The procedures were approved by the institutional review board of the University of Washington. All participants provided written informed consent and received $20 for completing the study.

Measures

Trauma exposure. The Traumatic Life Events Questionnaire (TLEQ; Kubany et al., 2000) is a self-report measure that assesses a broad range of potentially traumatic life events and has good psychometric properties. Participants were asked to indicate whether they had experienced potentially traumatic events during the following timeframes: (a) before they enlisted, (b) during active duty, or (c) after military service (as a Veteran). Although the TLEQ requests that respondents indicate whether they experienced PTSD Criterion A2 at the time of each traumatic event endorsed, we did not use this to determine trauma endorsement given its limited ability to predict PTSD symptoms (e.g., Kubany, Ralston, & Hill, 2010). A participant was considered to have been exposed to MSA if he or she endorsed experiencing the following during active duty: "After your 18th birthday: Did anyone touch sexual parts of your body or make you touch sexual parts of their body—against your will or without your consent?" The TLEQ was also used to examine childhood and other non-MSA adulthood interpersonal trauma. *Childhood interpersonal trauma* was defined as childhood sexual abuse either by someone at least 5 years older or without consent, sexual abuse during the teenage years, and childhood physical abuse, whereas *other non-MSA adulthood interpersonal trauma* was defined as adulthood sexual assault during pre- or post-military service and spousal physical abuse. The final question requested that respondents endorse which potentially traumatic life event of those that they had experienced currently caused them the most distress. The above noted timeframes were not associated with this question; thus, it is unclear when the endorsement of adulthood sexual assault occurred in reference to one's military service.

PTSD. The PTSD Checklist–Civilian version (Weathers, Litz, Herman, Huska, & Keane, 1993) is a well-validated 17-item self-report measure assessing the severity of PTSD symptomatology consistent with *Diagnostic and Statistical Manual of Mental Disorders* (4th ed.; *DSM–IV*) criteria. Items are measured on a 5-point Likert scale (1 = *not at all* to 5 = *extremely*). Scores range from 17 to 85, with higher values indicating greater psychopathology.

Depression. The Patient Health Questionnaire-9 (PHQ-9) (Kroenke, Spitzer, & Williams, 2001) is a validated 9-item self-report measure assessing the severity of depressive symptomatology consistent with *DSM–IV* criteria. Scores range from 0 to 27, and higher scores indicate greater depression.

DESNOS interview. The Structured Interview for Disorders of Extreme Stress (SIDES; van der Kolk et al., 1992; Zlotnick & Pearlstein, 1997) is a 48-item structured interview that assesses lifetime and current DESNOS. Pelcovitz et al. (1997) reported evidence of adequate interrater reliability and internal consistency for the SIDES total score in community and clinical samples. The present study focused on current DESNOS severity within the standard 1-month timeframe. Items are rated on a 4-point scale ranging from 0, indicating no problem, to 3, indicating extreme problems. Consistent with research using modifications of the scoring strategy for the SIDES (e.g., Ford et al., 2006; Zlotnick & Pearlstein, 1997), items were summed to obtain a severity score ranging from 0 to 135 (Cronbach's α total score for the present sample = .90).

Administrative database information. The VA VISN 20 data warehouse was used to identify the initial sample of 977 based on the inclusion criteria and to extract pertinent patient descriptive data.

RESULTS

Sample Characteristics

Descriptive statistics are presented separately in Table 1 for female and male Veterans because of gender differences in the prevalence of MSA in this sample. A majority (63.5%, $n = 66$) of female Veterans and a small minority (5.8%, $n = 6$) of male Veterans endorsed experiencing MSA. Given the small

TABLE 1 Demographic Characteristics Across Female and Male Veterans ($N = 208$)

Characteristic	Females	Males
Age, *M* (*SD*)	48.6 (9.8)	56.2 (11.3)
Ethnicity, %		
Caucasian	74	76
African American	10.6	14.4
Asian American	2.9	1.9
Hispanic	1.9	2.9
Marital status, %		
Married	40.4	46.2
Divorced/separated	40.4	33.7
Never married	17.3	17.3
Education: completed at least some college, %	54.8	50
VA service-connected disability, %		
At least 50% or greater	66.3	64.4
Less than 50%	17.3	15.4
Non-service connected	16.3	20.2
Annual household income above $25,000, %	56.7	55

Notes. VA = Veterans Affairs.

number of male Veterans in this sample who endorsed MSA, we chose to focus the remaining analyses on female Veterans, consistent with other studies that have lacked power to assess sequelae of MST in men (Surís & Lind, 2008).

Table 2 illustrates the type and frequency of trauma endorsement in this sample of female Veterans for those who did and did not endorse MSA, based on the lifetime trauma exposure categories on the TLEQ. Female Veterans who endorsed MSA reported greater numbers of other (non-MSA) potentially traumatic events during their lifetime ($M = 11.3$, $SD = 3.7$) compared to their peers without a history of MSA ($M = 9.4$, $SD = 4.2$), $t(102) = -2.4$, $p < .05$. Of those who endorsed experiencing MSA, a minority (females: 31.8%, $n = 21$; males: 16.7%, $n = 1$) indicated that unwanted sexual contact as an adult, the category that includes participants' MSA experiences, currently caused them the most distress compared to other potentially traumatic events.

Mental Health Correlates Associated with MSA

Zero-order correlations indicated that depression was significantly related to PTSD ($r = .77$, $p < .05$) and DESNOS ($r = .74$, $p < .05$). Given this significant association, depression was not explored in subsequent analyses. PTSD and DESNOS were also significantly associated with each other in this sample ($r = .71$, $p < .05$); however, we chose to retain them both in subsequent analyses given their conceptualization as trauma-specific psychological sequelae that have been shown to be independent of each other (Ford et al., 2006).

TABLE 2 Endorsement of Potentially Traumatic Events Among Female Veterans With and Without MSA

	Females ($N = 104$)					
	MSA ($N = 66$)			No MSA ($N = 38$)		
Trauma type	Before	During	After	Before	During	After
Natural disaster	53.0	40.9	69.7	52.6	23.7	57.9
Motor vehicle accident	21.2	25.8	34.8	31.6	18.4	39.5
Other accident	25.8	22.7	15.2	21.1	21.1	10.5
War zone	1.5	12.1	4.5	0.0	13.2	0.0
Death of a loved one	56.1	45.5	72.7	42.1	52.6	68.4
Loved one suffering	42.4	36.4	56.1	26.3	28.9	50.0
Personal illness	16.7	22.7	33.3	15.8	21.1	26.3
Robbery	16.7	13.6	10.6	2.6	2.6	7.9
Assault by stranger	21.2	30.3	13.6	15.8	13.2	18.4
Witnessed assault	18.2	18.2	7.6	10.5	7.9	2.6
Death threat	36.4	54.5	42.4	13.2	23.7	23.7
Childhood physical abuse	51.5			36.8		
Family violence	64.6[a]			47.2[b]		
Spousal physical abuse	24.2	39.4	33.3	21.1	18.4	21.1
CSA by an adult	61.5[a]			55.3		
CSA by peer	61.5[a]			55.3		
Teen sexual abuse	43.9			34.2		
Adult sexual assault	33.3	100.0	28.8	18.4	0.0	10.5
Sexual harassment	43.9	87.9	47.0	34.2	55.3	26.3
Stalking	9.1	43.9	37.9	10.5	15.8	28.9
Miscarriage	18.2	18.2	15.2	7.9	10.5	10.5
Abortion	9.1	19.7	13.6	15.8	15.8	13.2
Other	40.9	50.0	45.5	34.2	34.2	36.8

Notes. Data are percentages. MSA = military sexual assault; CSA = childhood sexual abuse.
[a]$N = 65$. [b]$N = 36$.

To examine the unique contribution that MSA has in predicting PTSD and DESNOS symptoms while taking into account childhood and other adulthood interpersonal trauma, we conducted hierarchical multiple regression analyses with Bonferroni corrections to control for multiple tests ($p < .05/2 = .025$). At Step 1, childhood interpersonal trauma variables were entered, with non-MSA adulthood interpersonal trauma variables entered at Step 2. MSA was entered on the final step. For the analysis examining PTSD, childhood interpersonal trauma predicted PTSD, $F(3, 97) = 3.33$, $p < .025$, and accounted for 9% of the variance; non-MSA adulthood interpersonal trauma accounted for an additional 6.5% of the unique variance (see Table 3). MSA captured 5.9% of the unique variance in predicting PTSD symptoms after both childhood and adulthood interpersonal trauma were taken into account. In predicting DESNOS symptoms, childhood interpersonal trauma accounted for 12% of the variance, $F(3, 100) = 4.33$, $p < .025$. In Step 2, non-MSA adulthood interpersonal trauma added an additional 4.1% of the unique variance, whereas MSA captured 6.6% of the unique variance in predicting DESNOS symptoms (see Table 4).

TABLE 3 Hierarchical Regression Analyses Examining Childhood and Adulthood Interpersonal Trauma and MSA in Predicting PTSD

Predictor	*B* (*SE*)	*β*	Partial *F*	*df*	R^2	Adjusted R^2	ΔR^2	*F* change
Step 1			3.33*	3,97	.09	.07	.09	3.33*
Childhood sexual abuse	2.95 (3.55)	.09						
Teen sexual abuse	−2.34 (3.58)	−.07						
Childhood physical abuse	9.47 (3.47)	.29*						
Step 2			2.95*	6,94	.16	.11	.07	2.42
Spousal physical abuse	−4.96 (3.20)	−.15						
Pre-MSA	−4.10 (3.87)	−.11						
Post-MSA	−7.43 (3.95)	−.19						
Step 3			3.70*	7,93	.22	.16	.06	7.07*
MSA	8.54 (3.21)	.25*						

Notes. MSA = military sexual assault; PTSD = posttraumatic stress disorder.
* $p < .025$.

TABLE 4 Hierarchical Regression Analyses Examining Childhood and Adulthood Interpersonal Trauma and MSA in Predicting DESNOS

Predictor	*B* (*SE*)	*β*	Partial *F*	*df*	R^2	Adjusted R^2	ΔR^2	*F* change
Step 1			4.33*	3,100	.12	.09	.12	4.33*
Childhood sexual abuse	4.59 (3.75)	.13						
Teen sexual abuse	2.57 (3.83)	.07						
Childhood physical abuse	8.47 (3.67)	.24*						
Step 2			2.99*	6,97	.16	.10	.04	1.58
Spousal physical abuse	−0.55 (3.43)	−.02						
Pre-MSA	0.70 (4.23)	.02						
Post-MSA	−9.28 (4.30)	−.22						
Step 3			3.91*	7,96	.22	.17	.07	8.09*
MSA	9.78 (3.44)	.27*						

Notes. MSA = military sexual assault; DESNOS = disorders of extreme stress not otherwise specified.
* $p < .025$.

Characteristics of Those Identifying Adult Sexual Assault as Most Distressing

The majority of females endorsing a history of MSA ($n = 45$, 68.2%) indicated that some other potentially traumatic event was currently most distressing and thereby more distressing than unwanted adult sexual contact. (Note that a differentiation could not be made between MSA and another unwanted adult sexual contact for this question.) Among women who reported MSA, those who reported adult sexual assault as currently most distressing evidenced greater PTSD ($M = 60.2$, $SD = 10.2$) compared to those who endorsed another potentially traumatic event as most distressing ($M = 51.39$, $SD = 15.34$), $t(63) = -2.40$, $p < .025$, with Bonferroni corrections for multiple comparisons (.05/2 = .025). DESNOS symptoms followed a similar pattern, as those who endorsed adult sexual assault as most distressing reported greater DESNOS symptoms ($M = 42.0$, $SD = 16.2$) when compared with those who did not ($M = 31.3$, $SD = 16.8$), $t(64) = -2.42$, $p < .025$.

DISCUSSION

The present study explored the posttraumatic sequelae associated with MSA in a sample of female Veterans engaged in VA outpatient mental health services. Consistent with previous findings (e.g., Himmelfarb et al., 2006; Surís et al., 2007), female Veterans who endorsed MSA evidenced increased PTSD and DESNOS symptoms as compared to their female counterparts without MSA. Regression analyses taking into account the impact of childhood and non-MSA adulthood interpersonal trauma found that MSA continues to partially predict PTSD and DESNOS symptoms, contributing 6% and 7% of the unique variance, respectively. Childhood interpersonal trauma also accounted for a clinically significant amount of the variance in predicting PTSD and DESNOS symptoms. Approximately a third of the female Veterans who endorsed MSA reported that they were currently most distressed by MSA relative to other potentially traumatic events, and they also reported greater PTSD and DESNOS symptoms than those who perceived another potentially traumatic event as most troubling.

The female Veterans within this sample reported a high rate of exposure to interpersonal trauma across the lifespan, consistent with other studies examining lifetime trauma prevalence in outpatient VA Medical Center samples (e.g., Polusny, Dickinson, Murdoch, & Thuras, 2008). In the context of significant interpersonal trauma exposure, MSA was associated with DESNOS symptomatology, which includes emotion regulation difficulties, interpersonal problems, dissociation, somatization, negative self-perception, and significant alterations in systems of meaning (e.g., hopelessness). Consistent with evidence suggesting an association between childhood interpersonal trauma and DESNOS (e.g., Ford, 1999; Ford et al., 2006; van der Kolk et al., 2005), this study found that childhood interpersonal trauma captured 12% of the unique variance in DESNOS symptoms, whereas MSA captured 7% of the unique variance when childhood and other adulthood interpersonal trauma were taken into account. Although we cannot determine causation with these cross-sectional data, our results suggest that MSA contributes important variance to DESNOS symptoms and that both of these types of interpersonal traumas are likely associated with DESNOS symptomatology. One significant clinical implication of the DESNOS construct is its association with poorer PTSD treatment outcome (Ford & Kidd, 1998). Therefore, treatments more likely to address DESNOS symptoms may be beneficial for this subset of Veterans who have experienced MSA. For example, clinicians and researchers (Cloitre, Koenen, Cohen, & Han, 2002; Courtois & Ford, 2009; Wagner & Linehan, 2006) have suggested a phase-based approach originally put forth by Herman (1992b) to address such complex posttraumatic reactions.

Despite the relationship between MSA and significant psychiatric symptoms reported by this VA mental health treatment–seeking sample (50% of which was involved in the Women's PTSD Careline), MSA was not the most troubling traumatic event reported for approximately two thirds of the women who reported MSA. These findings suggest that exposure to other potentially traumatic events should be assessed and considered in the treatment of women reporting MSA and suggest the possibility, untested in this study, that various factors such as recency of exposure to MSA may account for the endorsement of MSA as most troubling. A limitation of this study is the inability to examine MSA separately from civilian adulthood sexual assault in terms of the traumatic event that participants endorsed as currently most distressing. Despite this, those participants who did endorse adulthood sexual assault (including MSA) as currently most distressing endorsed more severe PTSD and DESNOS symptoms than those who reported another potentially traumatic event as most troubling. Thus, treatment addressing not only PTSD but also DESNOS symptoms is indicated for these female Veterans.

A limitation of this study is the use of an exclusively Veteran patient sample specifically enrolled in mental health service, as this limits the generalizability of the study findings to other populations and the ability to explore posttraumatic reactions to MSA in Veterans outside the VA system. The study's focus on treatment-seeking Veterans, however, provides a more detailed picture of the experiences and needs of female VA mental health patients, an identified population in need of further study. Another limitation is the loss of 23% of eligible participants considered too clinically unstable to participate as defined by their primary mental health practitioners, which may have skewed the data to not adequately capture these individuals. Additional limitations are the lack of systematic interrater reliability on the DESNOS interview, although ongoing supervision was done, and the limited psychometric research on the SIDES as a measure of DESNOS. Researchers have recently revised the SIDES, and the revised version has evidenced good psychometric properties in terms of both reliability and validity (Scoboria, Ford, Lin, & Frisman, 2008). Future research examining MST and DESNOS using this measure would be fruitful. This research was also limited in the cross-sectional, correlational nature of the data as well as in sample size, which limited our power to detect group differences in female Veterans and to explore posttraumatic sequelae associated with MSA in male Veterans. Future research would likely profit from larger scale investigations that capture a VA mental health treatment–seeking sample and from prospective designs.

This study found that in women seeking treatment in VA mental health clinics, the subjective current impact of MSA experiences varied across individuals. Our assessment of the relative contribution of MSA to the picture of psychopathology was clearly limited and provides very rudimentary information about the impact of MSA relative to other potential stressors. For instance, the PTSD self-report measure used in this study did not associate symptoms with a specific potentially traumatic event. Future research should explore the context and characteristics of MSA experiences and more thoroughly assess the relative impact of these stressful events on Veterans' psychosocial functioning.

Although preliminary, this study suggests that the DESNOS construct may be particularly relevant for female Veterans who report experiencing MSA. However, it is important that experts not remain focused on a simple association, as the picture of MSA is likely more complex, and its current role in Veterans' lives is clearly not uniform. Female Veterans with MSA seeking mental health treatment may range from those who exhibit more complex posttraumatic reactions (more severe PTSD, DESNOS, depression) to those who appear less bothered by past MSA experiences. Understanding the impact of specific contextual factors associated with a Veteran's MSA and other potentially traumatic events on posttraumatic reactions may provide for more targeted and therefore more effective treatment interventions as well as increased efficiency of VA mental health resources and greater patient satisfaction.

REFERENCES

Cloitre, M., Koenen, K. C., Cohen, L. R., & Han, H. (2002). Skills training in affective and interpersonal regulation followed by exposure: A phase-based treatment for PTSD related to childhood abuse. *Journal of Consulting and Clinical Psychology*, *70*, 1067–1074.

Courtois, C. A., & Ford, J. D. (2009). *Treating complex traumatic stress disorders: An evidence-based guide*. New York, NY: Guilford Press.

Engel, C. C., Engel, A. L., Campbell, S. J., McFall, M. E., Russo, J., & Katon, W. (1993). Posttraumatic stress disorder symptoms and precombat sexual and physical abuse in Desert Storm veterans. *Journal of Nervous and Mental Disease*, *181*, 683–688.

Fontana, A., & Rosenheck, R. (1998). Duty-related and sexual stress in the etiology of PTSD among women veterans who seek treatment. *Psychiatric Services*, *49*, 658–662.

Fontana, A., Schwartz, L., & Rosenheck, R. (1997). Posttraumatic stress disorder among female Vietnam veterans: A causal model of etiology. *American Journal of Public Health*, *87*, 169–175.

Ford, J. D. (1999). Disorders of extreme stress following war-zone military trauma: Associated features of posttraumatic stress disorder or comorbid but distinct syndromes? *Journal of Consulting and Clinical Psychology*, *67*, 3–12.

Ford, J. D., & Kidd, P. (1998). Early childhood trauma and disorders of extreme stress as predictors of treatment outcome with chronic posttraumatic stress disorder. *Journal of Traumatic Stress*, *11*, 743–761.

Ford, J. D., Stockton, P., Kaltman, S., & Green, B. L. (2006). Disorders of extreme stress (DESNOS) symptoms are associated with type and severity of interpersonal trauma exposure in a sample of healthy young women. *Journal of Interpersonal Violence*, *21*, 1399–1416.

Hankin, C., Skinner, K., Sullivan, L., Miller, D., Frayne, S., & Tripp, T. (1999). Prevalence of depressive and alcohol abuse symptoms among women VA outpatients who report experiencing sexual assault while in the military. *Journal of Traumatic Stress*, *12*, 601–612.

Herman, J. L. (1992a). Complex PTSD: A syndrome in survivors of prolonged and repeated trauma. *Journal of Traumatic Stress*, *5*, 377–391.

Herman, J. L. (1992b). *Trauma and recovery: The aftermath of violence—From domestic violence to political terror*. New York, NY: Basic Books.

Himmelfarb, N., Yaeger, D., & Mintz, J. (2006). Posttraumatic stress disorder in female veterans with military and civilian sexual trauma. *Journal of Traumatic Stress*, *19*, 837–846.

King, D. W., King, L. A., Foy, D. W., & Gudanowski, D. M. (1996). Prewar factors in combat-related posttraumatic stress disorder: Structural equation modeling with a national sample of female and male Vietnam veterans. *Journal of Consulting and Clinical Psychology*, *64*, 520–531.

King, D. W., King, L. A., Foy, D. W., Keane, T. M., & Fairbank, J. A. (1999). Posttraumatic stress disorder in a national sample of female and male Vietnam veterans: Risk factors, war-zone stressors, and resilience-recovery variables. *Journal of Abnormal Psychology*, *108*, 164–170.

Kroenke, K., Spitzer, R. L., & Williams, J. B. (2001). The PHQ-9 Validity of a brief depression severity measure. *Journal of Internal Medicine*, *16*, 606–613.

Kubany, E. S., Leisen, M. B., Kaplan, A. S., Watson, S. B., Haynes, S. N., Owens, J. A., & Burns, K. (2000). Development and preliminary validation of a brief broad-spectrum measure of trauma exposure: The Traumatic Life Events Questionnaire. *Psychological Assessment*, *12*, 210–224.

Kubany, E. S., Ralston, T. C., & Hill, E. E. (2010). Intense fear, helplessness, "and" horror? An empirical investigation of *DSM-IV* PTSD Criterion A2. *Psychological Trauma: Theory, Research, Practice, and Policy*, *2*, 77–82.

Murdoch, M., Polusny, M. A., Hodges, J., & O'Brien, N. (2004). Prevalence of in-service and post-service sexual assault among combat and noncombat veterans applying for Department of Veterans Affairs posttraumatic stress disorder disability benefits. *Military Medicine*, *169*, 392–395.

Pelcovitz, D., van der Kolk, B., Roth, S., Mandel, F., Kaplan, S., & Resick, P. (1997). Development of a criteria set and a structured interview for disorders of extreme stress (DESNOS). *Journal of Traumatic Stress*, *10*, 3–16.

Polusny, M. A., Dickinson, K. A., Murdoch, M., & Thuras, P. (2008). The role of cumulative sexual trauma and difficulties identifying feelings in understanding female veterans' physical health outcomes. *General Hospital Psychiatry*, *30*, 162–170.

Roth, S., Newman, E., Pelcovitz, D., van der Kolk, B., & Mandel, F. (1997). DESNOS in victims exposed to sexual/physical abuse. *Journal of Traumatic Stress*, *10*, 539–555.

Sadler, A. G., Booth, B. M., Mengeling, M. A., & Doebbeling, B. N. (2004). Life span and repeated violence against women during military service: Effects on health status and outpatient utilization. *Journal of Women's Health*, *13*, 799–811.

Scoboria, A., Ford, J., Lin, H., & Frisman, L. (2008). Exploratory and confirmatory factor analyses of the Structured Interview for Disorders of Extreme Stress. *Assessment*, *15*, 404–425.

Surís, A., & Lind, L. (2008). Military sexual trauma: A review of prevalence and associated health consequences in veterans. *Trauma, Violence, and Abuse*, *9*, 250–269.

Surís, A., Lind, L., Kashner, T. M., & Borman, P. D. (2007). Mental health, quality of life, and health functioning in women veterans: Differential outcomes associated with military and civilian sexual assault. *Journal of Interpersonal Violence*, *22*, 179–197.

Surís, A., Lind, L., Kashner, T. M., Borman, P. D., & Petty, F. (2004). Sexual assault in women veterans: An examination of PTSD risk, health care utilization, and cost of care. *Psychosomatic Medicine*, *66*, 749–756.

Valente, S., & Wright, C. (2007). Military sexual trauma: Violence and sexual abuse. *Military Medicine*, *172*, 259–265.

van der Kolk, B., Pelcovitz, D., Herman, J., Roth, S., Kaplan, S., & Spitzer, R. (1992). *Structured Interview for Disorders of Extreme Stress*. Unpublished manuscript.

van der Kolk, B. A., Roth, S., Pelcovitz, D., Sunday, S., & Spinazzola, J. (2005). Disorders of extreme stress: The empirical foundation of a complex adaptation to trauma. *Journal of Traumatic Stress*, *18*, 389–399.

Wagner, A. W., & Linehan, M. M. (2006). Applications of dialectical behavior therapy to posttraumatic stress disorder and related problems. In V. M. Follette & J. I. Rusek (Eds.), *Cognitive-behavioral therapies for trauma* (2nd ed., pp. 117–145). New York, NY: Guilford Press.

Weathers, F. W., Litz, B. T., Herman, D. S., Huska, J. A., & Keane, T. M. (1993, October). *The PTSD Checklist (PCL): Reliability, validity, and diagnostic utility*. Paper presented at the 9th Annual Meeting of the International Society for Traumatic Stress Studies, San Antonio, TX.

Wolfe, J., Sharkansky, E. J., Read, J. P., Dawson, R., Martin, J. A., & Ouimette, P. C. (1998). Sexual harassment and assault as predictors of PTSD symptomatology among U.S. female Persian Gulf War military personnel. *Journal of Interpersonal Violence*, *13*, 40–57.

Yaeger, D., Himmelfarb, N., Cammack, A., & Mitz, J. (2006). *DSM-IV* diagnosed posttraumatic stress disorder in women veterans with and without military sexual trauma. *Journal of General Internal Medicine*, *21*, S65–S69.

Zlotnick, C., & Pearlstein, T. (1997). Validation of the Structured Interview for Disorders of Extreme Stress. *Comprehensive Psychiatry*, *38*, 243–247.

Posttraumatic Stress Symptomatology as a Mediator of the Association Between Military Sexual Trauma and Post-Deployment Physical Health in Women

BRIAN N. SMITH, PhD and JILLIAN C. SHIPHERD, PhD

Women's Health Sciences Division, National Center for PTSD, VA Boston Healthcare System, Boston, Massachusetts, USA; and Boston University School of Medicine, Boston, Massachusetts, USA

JENNIFER L. SCHUSTER, PhD

Women's Health Sciences Division, National Center for PTSD, VA Boston Healthcare System, Boston, Massachusetts, USA

DAWNE S. VOGT, PhD

Women's Health Sciences Division, National Center for PTSD, VA Boston Healthcare System, Boston, Massachusetts, USA; and Boston University School of Medicine, Boston, Massachusetts, USA

LYNDA A. KING, PhD

Women's Health Sciences Division, National Center for PTSD, VA Boston Healthcare System Boston, Massachusetts, USA; and Departments of Psychiatry and Psychology, Boston University, Boston, Massachusetts, USA

DANIEL W. KING, PhD

Behavioral Science Division, National Center for PTSD, VA Boston Healthcare System, Boston, Massachusetts, USA; and Departments of Psychiatry and Psychology, Boston University, Boston, Massachusetts, USA

This study was supported by a Department of Defense/Department of Veterans Affairs grant ("Measurement and Validation of Psychosocial Risk and Resilience Factors Associated With Physical and Mental Health-Related Quality of Life in Persian Gulf War Veterans," PG Project DoD-87, Daniel W. King and Lynda A. King, co-principal investigators). The authors also thank the National Center for PTSD for ongoing support.

This study examined posttraumatic stress symptomatology (PSS) as a mediator of the association between military sexual trauma and post-deployment physical health. Relationships were examined in a sample of 83 female veterans of the first Gulf War (1990–1991) approximately 10 years post-deployment. Participants reported on the frequency of sexual harassment and sexual assault experienced during deployment. Physical health was measured using participants' self-reports of pre-deployment and post-deployment symptoms within 7 body systems. Sexual harassment exposure was not found to be associated with PSS-mediated associations with physical health symptoms. However, sexual assault during deployment was found to be associated with PSS and 4 of the 7 health symptom clusters assessed: gastrointestinal, genitourinary, musculoskeletal, and neurological symptoms. Furthermore, PSS was found to be a significant mediator of the sexual assault–physical health relationship in each of these domains, with the indirect path accounting for 74% to 100% of the relationship. The findings from the current study indicate that sexual assault has detrimental associations with physical health and that PSS plays a primary role in that relationship.

Exposure to potentially traumatic events is associated with decrements in physical health (Ramchand, Marshall, Schell, & Jaycox, 2008; Sareen et al., 2007; Schnurr & Spiro, 1999; Vasterling et al., 2008; Wolfe, Schnurr, Brown, & Furey, 1994). However, exposure to potentially traumatic events alone is not sufficient to result in poor physical health, but rather trauma appears to precede mental health symptoms that could underlie later physical health issues. Posttraumatic stress disorder (PTSD) has been highlighted in leading theoretical models that argue that PTSD symptoms are the primary mechanism through which trauma results in poor physical health (Schnurr & Green, 2004a, 2004b; Schnurr & Jankowski, 1999). Indeed, several studies have reported findings that posttraumatic stress symptomatology (PSS) mediates—either partially or fully—the relationship between trauma exposure and poor physical health (Campbell, Greeson, Bybee, & Raja, 2008; Dutton et al., 2006; Jakupcak, Luterek, Hunt, Conybeare, & McFall, 2008; Lang et al., 2006, 2008). The aim of the present study was to examine the potential mediating role of PSS in the association between exposure to a particular type of stressor—military sexual trauma (MST)—and subsequent physical health symptomatology.

Associations between stress reactions and physical health are seen across a number of domains, including cardiovascular, respiratory, gastrointestinal, cancer, and chronic pain problems (e.g., Sareen et al., 2007). Schnurr, Spiro, and Paris (2000) found that war zone stressor–related PSS was associated with increased onset of disordered functioning in several body systems, including the arterial, gastrointestinal, and musculoskeletal systems. Significant associations were also found between PTSD and several physical health indices in soldiers 1 year post-deployment (Hoge, Terhakopian, Castro, Messer, & Engel, 2007). It is important that even after demographic factors and comorbid mental health complaints are controlled, PSS appears to demonstrate a unique contribution to physical health symptoms (e.g., Jakupcak et al., 2008).

Although there is empirical support for the association between PSS and physical health outcomes, these relationships may differ between men and women. Differences in the rates and types of trauma exposure as well as differing rates of some physical illnesses could be salient. Therefore, studies that examine sex differences or assess associations for men and women separately are needed. Norman and colleagues (2006) examined associations between psychological trauma and physical illness in a sample of male and female primary care patients and tested whether a diagnosis of PTSD would mediate these associations. For men, PTSD mediated the trauma exposure–health relationship for only one of nine illnesses, and no PTSD mediation was found for women. The authors suggested that PSS, rather than PTSD diagnosis, may mediate the relationship between trauma exposure and health outcomes, and they recommended further research.

Although exact prevalence rates of MST are not known, the Department of Defense conservatively estimates that 9% of active duty women experience sexual assault (unwanted physical sexual contact) and 52% endorse sexual harassment, including sexual behaviors that create an intimidating or offensive work environment (Lipari, Cook, Rock, & Matos, 2008). Sexual harassment can include requests for sexual favors, remarks about an individual's sexual activities, and threats of retaliation for not being sexually cooperative; sexual assault can range from attempts to stroke or fondle to completed rape. Given the stigma and fear associated with endorsing sexual harassment and assault, the annual prevalence estimates cited above are widely considered underestimations.

In studies of Gulf War veterans, military sexual harassment and assault have been found to be associated with increases in mental health symptoms (Vogt, Pless, King, & King, 2005), even when combat exposure is controlled (Kang, Dalager, Mahan, & Ishii, 2005). Furthermore, soldiers and Veterans Affairs (VA) patients who endorse MST have increased physical health complaints and diagnoses (Frayne, Skinner, Sullivan, & Freund, 2003; Frayne et al., 1999; Martin, Rosen, Durand, Knudson, & Stretch, 2000; Sadler, Booth, Mengeling, & Doebbeling, 2004; Sadler, Booth, Nielson, & Doebbeling, 2000). It is important to note that MST occurs in a unique context of military service, which is simultaneously an employment, residential, and social context (Street, Vogt, & Dutra, 2009; Suris & Lind, 2008). As a result, these experiences may be especially detrimental to mental health, as evidenced by the findings of one study in which sexual trauma during military service was more strongly associated with PTSD than were civilian sexual trauma exposures (Himmelfarb, Yaeger, & Mintz, 2006).

Although it is widely accepted that MST experiences are associated with increases in PTSD (Fontana & Rosenheck, 1998; Kang et al., 2005; Kimerling, Gima, Smith, Street, & Frayne, 2007; Murdoch, Polusny, Hodges, & Cowper, 2006; Suris, Lind, Kashner, Borman, & Petty, 2004; Wolfe et al., 1998; Yaeger, Himmelfarb, Cammack, & Mintz, 2006), the role of PSS in the MST–physical health relationship is a relatively underexplored area. One study of female VA patients with heterogeneous trauma exposure, including sexual assault, found that PSS fully mediated the relationship between violence and physical health symptoms (Campbell et al., 2008). To our knowledge, only one study has examined the mediational role of PSS in the context of MST specifically (Shipherd, Pineles, Gradus, & Resick, 2009). This longitudinal study found that PSS mediated the relationship between MST and perceived physical health in men but not in women. However, it is important to note that participants were responding either in the immediate aftermath or while MST was ongoing (past 6 months). The authors posited that the participants might have been experiencing a "GI Jane" response in which an initial increase in physical fitness served a protective or coping function. It is not known how these findings might have differed if more time had elapsed between the MST and the assessment.

The current study is an examination of women who were deployed to the Gulf War. The mediational role of PSS on the associations between exposure to sexual harassment and assault and subsequent physical health symptomatology across several domains of health was examined. Associations between exposure to sexual harassment during deployment and physical health symptoms were expected to be at least partially mediated through PSS. Based on prior research implicating the role of stress reactions in the relationship between potentially traumatic events involving some degree of physical assault and physical health symptomatology (e.g., Campbell et al., 2008; Dutton et al., 2006), we hypothesized that PSS would fully mediate associations between sexual assault and physical health symptoms.

METHOD

Survey Procedure and Sample

For the purposes of this study, a sampling pool of 147 female Gulf War veterans from across the country was identified from a larger study (King, King, Bolton, Knight, & Vogt, 2008) that drew its sampling frame from the Defense Manpower Data Center and the VA Gulf War Health Registry. The current study was limited to female veterans, as the number of males endorsing MST in the larger project was too small to allow for an examination of the relationships between MST, PSS, and physical health. As approved by the VA Boston Healthcare System's institutional review board, veterans were first mailed a letter explaining the purpose of the study and ensuring confidentiality. Next, study measures were sent to potential participants, followed by a reminder card, a remailing of surveys to nonrespondents, and a final reminder card. The response rate for women was 56% ($N = 83$), once participants who could not be found by the postal service were considered. Participants provided information on sexual harassment and assault during deployment, PSS, and physical health symptoms. In this sample, 40.2% reported at least one incident of sexual harassment, 28% reported at least one incident of sexual assault, and 24% reported both experiences (note that these were not mutually exclusive groups). See Table 1 for additional demographic and military characteristics.

Measures

Exposure to sexual harassment and sexual assault during deployment. The sexual harassment scale from the Deployment Risk and Resilience Inventory (King, King, Vogt, Knight, & Samper, 2006) assessed sexual harassment (4 items) and sexual assault (3 items) during deployment. For each item, the participant was asked to indicate the frequency of harassment or assault by unit members or leaders during deployment on a 4-point scale ranging from 1 (*never*) to 4 (*many times*). The sexual harassment items

TABLE 1 Participant Demographic Characteristics

Characteristic	*n*	%
Race		
African American	19	26
White	54	74
Hispanic ethnicity		
Hispanic	14	16.9
Not Hispanic	69	83.1
Military branch		
Air Force	6	7.3
Army	71	86.6
Navy	5	6.1
Enlisted status		
Enlisted	62	78.5
Officer	17	21.5
Pre-deployment duty status		
Active duty	22	27.5
National Guard	14	17.5
Reserves	44	55
Age		
29–39	48	58
40–49	26	31
50–59	9	11

were as follows: "gossiped about my sex life or spread rumors about my sexual activities," "made crude and offensive sexual remarks directed at me, either publicly or privately," "threatened me with some sort of retaliation for not being sexually cooperative (for example, the threat of a negative review, physical violence, or to ruin my reputation, etc.)," and "offered me some sort of reward or special treatment to take part in sexual behavior." The sexual assault items were as follows: "made unwanted attempts to stroke or fondle me," "made unwanted attempts to have sex with me," and "forced me to have sex." Items were summed separately for sexual harassment and sexual assault during deployment.

PSS. PSS was assessed using the military version of the PTSD Checklist (Blanchard, Jones-Alexander, Buckley, & Forneris, 1996; Weathers, Litz, Herman, Huska, & Keane, 1993), a 17-item scale corresponding to the symptom criteria for PTSD based on the *Diagnostic and Statistical Manual of Mental Disorders* (4th ed.; American Psychiatric Association, 1994, 2000). Participants reported how much over the past 3 months they had been bothered by each symptom on a 5-point scale ranging from 1 (*not at all*) to 5 (*extremely*), with total scores used in the analyses. This scale was not used to determine PTSD diagnosis but rather level of symptoms. The measure has high internal consistency ($\alpha = .94$) and good test–retest reliability ($r = .96$, with a 2- to 3-day interval; Ruggiero, Del-Ben, Scotti, & Rabalais, 2003). The coefficient alpha for the PTSD Checklist in our sample was .95.

Physical health symptoms. A list of physical health symptoms was compiled based on a literature review of health problems reported by Gulf War veterans (Fukuda et al., 1998; Haley, 1997; Iowa Persian Gulf Study Group, 1997). Participants used a yes/no format to indicate health symptoms experienced both before deployment and after deployment. The dependent variable was a count of physical health symptoms occurring anytime post-deployment (past 10 years), and pre-deployment health symptoms counts were control variables. Following Proctor et al.'s (1998) classification scheme, we grouped each health symptom item into one of seven categories: cardiovascular (1 item), dermatological (2 items), gastrointestinal (3 items), genitourinary (2 items), musculoskeletal (5 items), neurological (7 items), and pulmonary (3 items). Items were summed within each category.

Exposure to warfare stressors. A composite of two Deployment Risk and Resilience Inventory scales assessing combat experiences and exposure to the aftermath of battle was completed by participants. Each scale consisted of 15 items and used a dichotomous (yes/no) response format. The combat experiences scale included traditional combat items (e.g., whether respondents were fired on by enemy), and the aftermath of battle scale included consequences of warfare (e.g., observing or handling human and animal remains). Because we were interested in controlling for the effect of the full range of warfare experiences, these scales were combined into one warfare exposure variable, consistent with prior studies (Vogt & Tanner, 2007).

Analyses

Sexual harassment and sexual assault during deployment were analyzed separately using SPSS Version 17.0. An outcome variable was considered significantly skewed if its skewness statistic exceeded twice its standard error (Hopkins & Weeks, 1990). PSS scores were positively skewed, and musculoskeletal symptoms were negatively skewed. A square root transformation increased the normality of PSS, whereas musculoskeletal symptoms were transformed using a reflect and square root transformation via the formula $\sqrt{(K - X)}$, where K is a constant equal to the largest score plus 1 (Tabachnick & Fidell, 1996). Bivariate correlations were used to examine the relationships among all variables (see Table 2). Potential confounding variables (i.e., race/ethnicity, age, and active duty/reserve status) were also examined via correlations with outcome variables. Effect sizes were interpreted using Cohen's (1988) guidelines.

Pre-deployment symptoms for each physical health cluster and exposure to warfare stressors were controlled for in the mediational analyses. When significant associations between sexual harassment or sexual assault and physical health symptoms were found, we tested our hypothesis that these relationships were mediated by PSS. The significance of mediated pathways was tested directly using the asymmetric distribution of products tests, as described by MacKinnon and colleagues (MacKinnon, Fritz, Williams, & Lockwood, 2007; MacKinnon, Lockwood, Hoffman, West, & Sheets, 2002). One regression was run to calculate the coefficient predicting the mediator from the independent variable (path a), controlling for covariates. If the first path was significant, a second regression was calculated predicting the outcome variable from the mediator (path b), controlling for the independent variable and covariates. Associated asymmetric confidence intervals were then calculated to test the significance of the indirect effect using the PRODCLIN program (MacKinnon, Fritz, et al., 2007). Effects were considered significant if

TABLE 2 Correlations Between PSS, Sexual Harassment, Sexual Assault, and Physical Health Symptoms

Variable	1	2	3	4	5	6	7	8	9	10
1. Sexual assault	—	.76*	.38*	.07	.20	.34*	.24*	24*	.32*	.17
2. Sexual harassment		—	.24*	.06	.09	.22*	.09	12	.23*	.03
3. PSS			—	.37*	.43*	.61*	.39*	48*	.62*	.34*
4. Cardiovascular				—	.26*	.45*	.31*	38*	.50*	.52*
5. Dermatological					—	.45*	.30*	42*	.44*	.47*
6. Gastrointestinal						—	.43*	45*	.63*	.51*
7. Genitourinary							—	33*	.38*	.35*
8. Musculoskeletal								—	.70*	.51*
9. Neurological									—	.47*
10. Pulmonary										—

Notes. PSS = posttraumatic stress symptomatology.
*$p < .05$.

the 95% confidence limits of the indirect effects did not include zero. Percent mediation was used as an index of effect size, calculated as the amount of the total relationship between the predictor and outcome variable (c pathway) that was accounted for by the indirect (a × b) pathway.

RESULTS

No significant correlations were found between demographic variables and deployment sexual harassment, sexual assault, or PSS. Age was positively correlated with musculoskeletal symptoms ($r = .23$, $p < .05$) and was therefore included as a covariate in the mediational analyses predicting musculoskeletal symptoms.

Significant positive correlations were noted between PSS and all post-deployment physical health clusters in the expected directions (see Table 2). Sexual harassment was significantly correlated with gastrointestinal and neurological symptoms post-deployment. Sexual assault was related to gastrointestinal, genitourinary, musculoskeletal, and neurological symptoms. No significant relationships were observed between MST variables and dermatological, cardiovascular, and pulmonary symptoms. All of the significant associations were in the hypothesized direction, such that greater exposure to sexual harassment and assault was associated with more physical health symptoms post-deployment.

In assessing mediation, we found that sexual harassment was not a significant predictor of PSS when warfare stressors were included in the regression (unstandardized coefficient = .07, $t = 1.25$, $p > .05$). Given that the relationship between the predictor and mediator (path a) was not significant, mediation was not supported (MacKinnon, Fairchild, & Fritz, 2007). Sexual assault was a significant predictor of PSS, even after we controlled for warfare stressors (unstandardized coefficient = .24, $t = 2.60$, $p < .05$). For physical health symptoms associated with sexual assault (gastrointestinal, genitourinary, musculoskeletal, and neurological), PSS mediated the relationship between sexual assault and health symptoms (see Table 3).[1] For each symptom cluster, c′ did not differ significantly from zero and the a × b path was statistically significant, together providing support that the indirect effect involving PSS was significant. PSS mediated 74% of the total relationship of sexual assault with gastrointestinal symptoms, 75% of the relationship with genitourinary symptoms, 100% of the relationship with musculoskeletal symptoms, and 92% of the relationship with neurological symptoms. Given that many of those reporting exposure to military sexual assault also reported exposure to sexual harassment, supplemental analyses were conducted to examine whether the observed associations between sexual assault, PSS, and physical health symptoms would remain when harassment was included in the same regressions. The results revealed the same pattern of significant findings as observed in the primary analyses.

TABLE 3 Summary of Mediation Tests with Sexual Assault as the Predictor, PSS as the Potential Mediator, and Post-Deployment Health Symptom Clusters as the Outcomes

	Regression analyses			95% CI		
Tested dependent variable	*B*	*t*	Wald	LL	UL	% Mediation
Gastrointestinal symptom cluster						
Path a: Sexual assault to PSS	.24*	2.60				
Path b: PSS to symptom cluster	.33*		19.24			
Direct path c′	.03		.21			
Indirect path a × b	.08*			.02	.16	74
Genitourinary symptom cluster						
Path a: Sexual assault to PSS	.24*	2.60				
Path b: PSS to symptom cluster	.23*		5.39			
Direct path c′	.04		.21			
Indirect path a × b	.05*			.01	.13	75
Musculoskeletal symptom cluster						
Path a: Sexual assault to PSS	.24*	2.60				
Path b: PSS to symptom cluster	.13*		7.44			
Direct path c′	.00		.00			
Indirect path a × b	.03*			.01	.07	100
Neurological symptom cluster						
Path a: Sexual assault to PSS	.24*	2.60				
Path b: PSS to symptom cluster	.24*		26.43			
Direct path c′	.01		.01			
Indirect path a × b	.06*			.01	.11	92

Notes. Linear regression was used in analyses predicting PSS; Poisson regression was used in analyses predicting physical health symptom clusters. PSS = posttraumatic stress symptomatology; CI = confidence interval; LL = lower limit; UL = upper limit.
$^*p < .05$.

DISCUSSION

The present study found that PSS mediated the relationship between sexual assault during deployment and physical health as reported 10 years post-deployment in the following domains: gastrointestinal, genitourinary, musculoskeletal, and neurological. In examining the relationship between sexual assault and physical health, we found that PSS played a key role, with the mediated pathway accounting for 74% to 100% of the trauma exposure–physical health symptomatology relationship. It is interesting that symptoms captured in the gastrointestinal cluster (e.g., frequent abdominal pain), the musculoskeletal cluster (e.g., muscle or joint pain), the genitourinary cluster (e.g., sexual discomfort or difficulties), and the neurological cluster (e.g., recurrent headaches) were primarily complaints related to chronic pain and were the only symptoms significantly related to sexual assault exposure, with the relationships all mediated by PSS. This pattern is consistent with prior research implicating PSS as a mediator of the relationship between exposure to interpersonal violence and physical health symptoms involving pain-related complaints (e.g., Campbell et al., 2008). In contrast, symptom clusters that did not include pain complaints (i.e., cardiovascular, dermatological, and pulmonary) were not significantly associated with deployment sexual harassment or assault. Although it is beyond the scope of this study to determine, perhaps the autoimmune response, as suggested by Campbell and colleagues (2008), is a key factor in these PSS-mediated effects. The larger literature on the association between chronic pain and PSS suggests that the current findings warrant further elaboration (Campbell et al., 2008; Otis, Keane, Kerns, Monson, & Scioli, 2009; Shipherd, Beck, Hamblen, Lackner, & Freeman, 2003; Shipherd et al., 2007).

Sexual harassment was significantly correlated with PSS as well as gastrointestinal and neurological symptoms at the bivariate level. However, PSS mediation of the relationships was not supported. It is unclear how to interpret the different pattern of findings with sexual harassment and assault, but it has been argued that these are qualitatively different stressors (e.g., Wolfe et al., 1998), though it is worth noting that many of those endorsing sexual assault also endorsed sexual harassment. Although both sexual harassment and sexual assault have been found to be related to deleterious health outcomes, studies have reported that associations with health decrements are stronger for sexual assault than sexual harassment (e.g., Street, Stafford, Mahan, & Hendricks, 2008), which is consistent with these data. A possible distinction between the stressors could be the physical nature of sexual assault. Perhaps the violent nature of the stressor is salient to sequelae. Furthermore, it is possible that the effects of sexual harassment are manifested in other negative ways (e.g., undermining the quality of relationships, self-image, and esteem) that were not examined in the current study. Though sexual harassment was not found to predict PSS after warfare stressors were controlled in this sample, it is important to further study the negative effects of such experiences.

The results of this study should be considered in light of some of the study's limitations. The cross-sectional nature of the study limits our ability to infer causality among the paths tested. Retrospective reporting of physical health, exposure to military sexual harassment and assault, and PSS is also a limitation. Though deployment-associated stress symptoms were likely in place for an extended period of time, it is possible that in some cases physical health symptoms may have preceded PSS. Assessing the constructs of interest at time points that align directly with the anticipated sequence of the hypothesized causal pathways, preferably in a longitudinal design, would further advance experts' understanding of these mechanisms. It should also be noted that the sample size for the present study was not large, which could have reduced our power to detect findings. However, even with this modest sample, significant indirect effects were found for sexual assault and PSS for multiple body systems. Replicating these findings in a larger sample would further improve confidence in the results as well as possibly facilitate the detection of weaker effects. Finally, it is important to acknowledge that men also experience MST, and some research suggests that men may have even more serious mental health consequences following MST than women (Kang et al., 2005; Shipherd et al., 2009; Street, Gradus, Stafford, & Kelly, 2007; Vogt et al., 2005). Future research would do well to investigate these relationships in both men and women, including an examination of sex differences when feasible.

Overall, the findings from the current study are consistent with the larger literature suggesting that stress exposure has detrimental effects on physical health and that PSS plays an important role in that relationship (Campbell et al., 2008; Dutton et al., 2006; Lang et al., 2006, 2008; Schnurr & Green, 2004a, 2004b; Schnurr & Jankowski, 1999). Future research should not only further examine the health consequences of MST and the pathways through which health is compromised but also assess the devastating long-term and potentially multiplicative effects of sexual harassment, sexual assault, and war zone–related stressors on health. Examining the consequences of sexual harassment and sexual assault represents an important research area, and more research is clearly needed, particularly given the prevalence of these traumatic stressors in both civilian and military environments.

NOTE

1. Approximately half of the participants from the current sample also responded to items assessing alcohol use and depression. Additional mediational analyses were tested for this subgroup controlling for depression and alcohol use, and the results, although only based on a subsample did mirror the findings of the larger study, such that including these additional variables as covariates yielded the same pattern of significant findings observed in the primary analyses on sexual assault. However, in the interest of preserving statistical power, the study sample was not limited to just those individuals who completed these additional measures.

REFERENCES

American Psychiatric Association. (1994). *Diagnostic and statistical manual of mental disorders* (4th ed.). Washington, DC: Author.

American Psychiatric Association. (2000). *Diagnostic and statistical manual of mental disorders* (4th ed., text rev.). Washington, DC: Author.

Blanchard, E. B., Jones-Alexander, J., Buckley, T. C., & Forneris, C. A. (1996). Psychometric properties of the PTSD Checklist (PCL). *Behaviour Research and Therapy*, *34*, 669–673.

Campbell, R., Greeson, M. R., Bybee, D., & Raja, S. (2008). The co-occurrence of childhood sexual abuse, adult sexual assault, intimate partner violence, and sexual harassment: A mediational model of posttraumatic stress disorder and physical health outcomes. *Journal of Consulting and Clinical Psychology, 76*, 194–207.

Cohen, J. (1988). *Statistical power analysis for the behavioral sciences* (2nd ed.). Hillsdale, NJ: Erlbaum.

Dutton, M. A., Green, B. L., Kaltman, S. I., Roesch, D. M., Zeffiro, T. A., & Krause, E. D. (2006). Intimate partner violence, PTSD, and adverse health outcomes. *Journal of Interpersonal Violence, 21*, 955–968.

Fontana, A., & Rosenheck, R. (1998). Duty-related and sexual stress in the etiology of PTSD among women veterans who seek treatment. *Psychiatric Services, 49*, 658–662.

Frayne, S., Skinner, K. M., Sullivan, L. M., & Freund, K. M. (2003). Sexual assault while in the military: Violence as a predictor of cardiac risk? *Violence and Victims, 18*, 219–225.

Frayne, S., Skinner, K. M., Sullivan, L. M., Tripp, T. J., Hankin, C. S., Kressin, N., & Miller, D. R. (1999). Medical profile of women Veterans Administration outpatients who report a history of sexual assault occurring while in the military. *Journal of Women's Health and Gender-Based Medicine, 8*, 835–845.

Fukuda, K., Nisenbaum, R., Stewart, G., Thompson, W. W., Robin, L., Washko, R. M., . . . Reeves, W. C. (1998). Chronic multisymptom illness affecting Air Force veterans of the Gulf War. *Journal of the American Medical Association, 280*, 981–988.

Haley, R. W. (1997). Is Gulf War syndrome due to stress? The evidence reexamined. *American Journal of Epidemiology, 146*, 695–703.

Himmelfarb, N., Yaeger, D., & Mintz, J. (2006). Posttraumatic stress disorder in female veterans with military and civilian sexual trauma. *Journal of Traumatic Stress, 19*, 837–846.

Hoge, C. W., Terhakopian, A., Castro, C. A., Messer, S. C., & Engel, C. C. (2007). Association of posttraumatic stress disorder with somatic symptoms, health care visits, and absenteeism among Iraq War veterans. *American Journal of Psychiatry, 164*, 150–153.

Hopkins, K. D., & Weeks, D. L. (1990). Tests for normality and measures of skewness and kurtosis: Their place in research reporting. *Educational and Psychological Measurement, 50*, 717–729.

Iowa Persian Gulf Study Group. (1997). Self-reported illness and health status among Gulf War veterans: A population-based study. *Journal of the American Medical Association, 277*, 238–245.

Jakupcak, M., Luterek, J., Hunt, S., Conybeare, D., & McFall, M. (2008). Posttraumatic stress and its relationship to physical health functioning in a sample of Iraq and Afghanistan war veterans seeking postdeployment VA health care. *Journal of Nervous and Mental Disease, 196*, 425–428.

Kang, H., Dalager, N., Mahan, C., & Ishii, E. (2005). The role of sexual assault on the risk of PTSD among Gulf War veterans. *Annals of Epidemiology, 15*, 191–195.

Kimerling, R., Gima, K., Smith, M. W., Street, A., & Frayne, S. (2007). The Veterans Health Administration and military sexual trauma. *American Journal of Public Health, 97*, 2160–2166.

King, L. A., King, D. W., Bolton, E. E., Knight, J. A., & Vogt, D. S. (2008). Risk factors for mental, physical, and functional health in Gulf War veterans. *Journal of Rehabilitation Research and Development*, *45*, 395–408.

King, L., King, D., Vogt, D., Knight, J A., & Samper, R. (2006). Deployment Risk and Resilience Inventory: A collection of measures for studying deployment-related experiences of military personnel and veterans. *Military Psychology*, *18*, 89–120.

Lang, A. J., Aarons, G. A., Gearity, J., Laffaye, C., Satz, L., Dresselhaus, T. R., & Stein, M. (2008). Direct and indirect links between childhood maltreatment, posttraumatic stress disorder, and women's health. *Behavioral Medicine*, *33*, 125–135.

Lang, A. J., Laffaye, C., Satz, L. E., McQuaid, J. R., Malcarne, V. L., Dresselhaus, T. R., & Stein, M. B. (2006). Relationships among childhood maltreatment, PTSD, and health in female veterans in primary care. *Child Abuse and Neglect*, *30*, 1281–1292.

Lipari, R. N., Cook, P. J., Rock, L. M., & Matos, K. (2008). *Gender relations survey of active duty members*. Arlington, VA: Defense Manpower Data Center.

MacKinnon, D. P., Fairchild, A. J., & Fritz, M. S. (2007). Mediation analysis. *Annual Review of Psychology*, *58*, 593–614.

MacKinnon, D. P., Fritz, M. S., Williams, J., & Lockwood, C. M (2007). Distribution of the product confidence limits for the indirect effect: Program PRODCLIN. *Behavior Research Methods*, *39*, 384–389.

MacKinnon, D. P., Lockwood, C. M., Hoffman, J. M., West, S. G., & Sheets, V. (2002). A comparison of methods to test mediation and other intervening variable effects. *Psychological Methods*, *7*, 83–104.

Martin, L., Rosen, L. N., Durand, D., Knudson, K. H., & Stretch, R. H. (2000). Psychological and physical health effects of sexual assaults and nonsexual traumas among male and female United States Army soldiers. *Behavioral Medicine*, *26*, 23–33.

Murdoch, M., Polusny, M. A., Hodges, J., & Cowper, D. (2006). The association between in-service sexual harassment and post-traumatic stress disorder among Department of Veterans Affairs disability applicants. *Military Medicine*, *17*, 166–173.

Norman, S. B., Means-Christensen, A. J., Craske, M. G., Sherbourne, C. D., Roy-Byrne, P. P., & Stein, M. B. (2006). Associations between psychological trauma and physical illness in primary care. *Journal of Traumatic Stress*, *19*, 461–470.

Otis, J. D., Keane, T. M., Kerns, R. D., Monson, C., & Scioli, E. (2009). The development of an integrated treatment for veterans with comorbid chronic pain and posttraumatic stress disorder. *Pain Medicine*, *10*, 1300–1311.

Proctor, S. P., Heeren, T., White, R. F., Wolfe, J., Borgos, M. S., Davis, J. D., . . . Ozonoff, D. (1998). Health status of Persian Gulf War veterans: Self-reported symptoms, environmental exposures and the effect of stress. *International Journal of Epidemiology*, *27* 1000–1010.

Ramchand, R., Marshall, G. N., Schell, T. L., & Jaycox, L. H. (2008). Posttraumatic distress and physical functioning: A longitudinal study of injured survivors of community violence. *Journal of Consulting and Clinical Psychology*, *76*, 668–676.

Ruggiero, J., Del-Ben, K., Scotti, J. R., & Rabalais, A. E. (2003). Psychometric properties of the PTSD Checklist–Civilian version. *Journal of Traumatic Stress*, *16*, 495–502.

Sadler, A. G., Booth, B. M., Mengeling, M. A., & Doebbeling, B. N. (2004). Life span and repeated violence against women during military service: Effects on health status and outpatient utilization. *Journal of Women's Health*, *13*, 799–811.

Sadler, A. G., Booth, B. M., Nielson, D., & Doebbeling, B. N. (2000). Health-related consequences of physical and sexual violence: Women in the military. *Obstetrics and Gynecology*, *96*, 473–480.

Sareen, J., Cox, B. J., Stein, M. B., Afifi, T. O., Fleet, C., & Asmundson, G. J. (2007). Physical and mental comorbidity, disability, and suicidal behavior associated with posttraumatic stress disorder in a large community sample. *Psychosomatic Medicine*, *69*, 242–248.

Schnurr, P. P., & Green, B. L. (2004a). *Trauma and health: Physical health consequences of exposure to extreme stress*. Washington, DC: American Psychological Association.

Schnurr, P. P., & Green, B. L. (2004b). Understanding relationships among trauma, post-traumatic stress disorder, and health outcomes. *Advances in Mind-Body Medicine*, *20*, 18–29.

Schnurr, P. P., & Jankowski, M. K. (1999). Physical health and post-traumatic stress disorder: Review and synthesis. *Seminars in Clinical Neuropsychiatry*, *4*, 295–304.

Schnurr, P. P., & Spiro, A., III. (1999). Combat exposure, posttraumatic stress disorder symptoms, and health behaviors as predictors of self-reported physical health in older veterans. *Journal of Nervous and Mental Disease*, *187*, 353–359.

Schnurr, P. P., Spiro, A., III, & Paris, A. H. (2000). Physician-diagnosed medical disorders in relation to PTSD symptoms in older male military veterans. *Health Psychology*, *19*, 91–97.

Shipherd, J. C., Beck, J. G., Hamblen, J. L., Lackner, J. M., & Freeman, J. B. (2003). A preliminary examination of treatment for posttraumatic stress disorder in chronic pain patients: A case study. *Journal of Traumatic Stress*, *16*, 451–457.

Shipherd, J. C., Keyes, M., Jovanovic, T., Ready, D., Baltzell, D., Worley, V., . . . Duncan, E. (2007). PTSD treatment seeking veterans: What about comorbid chronic pain? *Journal of Rehabilitation Research and Development*, *44*, 153–166.

Shipherd, J. C., Pineles, S. L., Gradus, J. L., & Resick, P. A. (2009). Sexual harassment in the Marines, posttraumatic stress symptoms, and perceived health: Evidence for sex differences. *Journal of Traumatic Stress*, *22*, 3–10.

Street, A. E., Gradus, J. L., Stafford, J., & Kelly, K. (2007). Gender differences in experiences of sexual harassment: Data from a male-dominated environment. *Journal of Consulting and Clinical Psychology*, *75*, 464–474.

Street, A. E., Stafford, J., Mahan, C. M., & Hendricks, A. (2008). Sexual harassment and assault experienced by reservists during military service: Prevalence and health correlates. *Journal of Rehabilitation Research and Development*, *45*, 409–419.

Street, A. E., Vogt, D. S., & Dutra, L. (2009). A new generation of women veterans: Stressors faced by women deployed to Iraq and Afghanistan. *Clinical Psychology Review*, *29*, 685–694.

Suris, A., & Lind, L. (2008). Military sexual trauma: A review of prevalence and associated health consequences in veterans. *Trauma, Violence, and Abuse*, *9*, 250–269.

Suris, A., Lind, L., Kashner, M., Borman, P. D., & Petty, F. (2004). Sexual assault in women veterans: An examination of PTSD risk, health care utilization and cost of care. *Psychosomatic Medicine*, *66*, 749–756.

Tabachnick, B. G., & Fidell, L. S. (1996). *Using multivariate statistics* (3rd ed.). New York, NY: HarperCollins College.

Vasterling, J. J., Schumm, J., Proctor, S. P., Gentry, E., King, D. W., & King, L. A. (2008). Posttraumatic stress disorder and health functioning in a non-treatment seeking sample of Iraq war veterans: A prospective analysis. *Journal of Rehabilitation Research and Development*, *45*, 347–358.

Vogt, D. S., Pless, A. P., King, L. A., & King, D. W. (2005). Deployment stressors, gender and mental health outcomes among Gulf War I veterans. *Journal of Traumatic Stress*, *18*, 115–127.

Vogt, D. S., & Tanner, L. R. (2007). Risk and resilience factors for posttraumatic stress symptomatology in Gulf War I veterans. *Journal of Traumatic Stress*, *20*(1), 27–38.

Weathers, F., Litz, B. T., Herman, D. S., Huska, J. A., & Keane, T. M. (1993, October). *The PTSD Checklist (PCL): Reliability, validity, and diagnostic utility*. Paper presented at the International Society for Traumatic Stress Studies, San Antonio, TX.

Wolfe, J., Schnurr, P. P., Brown, P. J., & Furey, J. (1994). Posttraumatic stress disorder and war-zone exposure as correlates of perceived health in female Vietnam War veterans. *Journal of Consulting and Clinical Psychology*, *62*, 1235–1240.

Wolfe, J., Sharkansky, E. J., Read, J. P., Dawson, R., Martin, J. A., Martin, J. A., & Oimette, P. C. (1998). Sexual harassment and assault as predictors of PTSD symptomatology among U.S. female Persian Gulf War military personnel. *Journal of Interpersonal Violence*, *13*, 40–57.

Yaeger, D., Himmelfarb, N., Cammack, A., & Mintz, J. (2006). *DSM-IV* diagnosed posttraumatic stress disorder in women veterans with and without military sexual trauma. *Journal of General Internal Medicine*, *21*(Suppl. 3), S65–S69.

Is Military Sexual Trauma Associated with Trading Sex Among Women Veterans Seeking Outpatient Mental Health Care?

JENNIFER L. STRAUSS, PhD

Health Services Research & Development, Durham VA Medical Center, Durham, North Carolina; Duke University Medical Center, Durham, North Carolina; and VA Mid-Atlantic Mental Illness Research, Education and Clinical Center, Durham, North Carolina, USA

CHRISTINE E. MARX, MD, MA

Duke University Medical Center, Durham, North Carolina; and VA Mid-Atlantic Mental Illness Research, Education and Clinical Center, Durham, North Carolina, USA

JULIE C. WEITLAUF, PhD

Sierra Pacific Mental Illness Research Education and Clinical Center, VA Palo Alto Health Care System, Menlo Park, California; Center for Health Care Evaluation, VA Palo Alto Health Care System, Menlo Park, California; VA Palo Alto Health Care System, Palo Alto, California; and Stanford University School of Medicine, Stanford, California, USA

KAREN M. STECHUCHAK, MS

Health Services Research & Development, Durham VA Medical Center, Durham, North Carolina, USA

KRISTY STRAITS-TRÖSTER, PhD

Duke University Medical Center, Durham, North Carolina; and VA Mid-Atlantic Mental Illness Research, Education and Clinical Center, Durham, North Carolina, USA

Dr. Butterfield died on June 26, 2006, after a courageous 5-year battle with breast cancer. The authors would like to acknowledge her work on the research described in this report and celebrate her many significant contributions to the field of psychiatry and the care of the nation's veterans. They would also like to acknowledge the hard work of Ms. Patricia Spivey and Dr. Mary Becker in gathering these data and Ms. Susan O'Loughlin in assisting with literature searches and manuscript formatting. This study was partially funded by Department of Veteran Affairs Research Career Development Awards to Jennifer L. Strauss, Christine E. Marx, Julie C. Weitlauf, and Marian I. Butterfield. The views expressed in this manuscript are those of the authors and do not necessarily represent the views of the Department of Veterans Affairs.

AYABA W. WORJOLOH, MD, MPH
Duke University School of Medicine, Durham, North Carolina; and Department of Obstetrics, Gynecology and Reproductive Sciences, University of California, San Francisco, San Francisco, California, USA

CHRISTINA B. SHERROD, PhD
VA Mid-Atlantic Mental Illness Research, Education and Clinical Center, Durham, North Carolina, USA

MAREN K. OLSEN, PhD
Health Services Research & Development, Durham VA Medical Center, Durham, North Carolina; and Duke University Medical Center, Durham, North Carolina, USA

MARIAN I. BUTTERFIELD, MD, MPH
and PATRICK S. CALHOUN, PhD
Health Services Research & Development, Durham VA Medical Center, Durham, North Carolina; Duke University Medical Center, Durham, North Carolina; and VA Mid-Atlantic Mental Illness Research, Education and Clinical Center, Durham, North Carolina, USA

A robust association between sexual trauma and trading sex has been documented in civilian samples but has not been examined in veterans. Women veterans experience high rates of sexual victimization across the lifespan, including during military service (military sexual trauma [MST]). Associations between MST and trading sex were examined in 200 women enrolled in a cross-sectional study of HIV risks and seroprevalence among women receiving outpatient mental health care at a Veterans Affairs (VA) medical center. Each woman completed an assessment interview composed of validated measures that queried childhood sexual trauma; substance use; and risk behaviors, including trading sex for money, drugs, shelter, food, or other things. History of MST was derived from mandated VA screening results and chart notes. Overall, 19.7% reported a history of trading sex. Those who reported trading sex had a higher rate of MST than those who did not report trading sex (87.2% vs. 62.9%, respectively). A multivariable logistic regression model examined the relationship between trading sex and MST, controlling a priori for substance abuse and childhood sexual trauma (both associated with trading sex in civilian samples) and education, which was associated with trading sex in our sample. In this adjusted model, MST was associated with trading sex: odds ratio = 3.26, p = .025, 95% confidence interval = [1.16, 9.18]. To our knowledge, this is the 1st report of an association between MST and trading sex. Results extend previously observed associations between sexual trauma and trading sex in civilian cohorts and underscore the pernicious influence of sexual victimization across the lifespan.

Exposure to sexual victimization has been linked with a broad array of adverse medical outcomes and complaints, including a greater incidence of gynecological disease and sexually transmitted infections (Dobie et al., 2004; Frayne, Skinner, Sullivan, & Freund, 2003; Letourneau, Holmes, & Chasedunn-Roark, 1999; Reynolds, Peipert, & Collins, 2000). Sexual victimization has also been linked with significant mental health consequences, including the development of mood disorders (e.g., depression and anxiety; Suris & Lind, 2008), substance use disorders, and posttraumatic stress disorder (PTSD; Dobie et al., 2004; Suris & Lind, 2008) and a greater likelihood of engaging in high-risk sexual behaviors (Burnette et al., 2008) that may intensify medical or mental health problems. For example, exposure to early (e.g., childhood), chronic (e.g., revictimization throughout the lifespan), or severe instances of sexual violence has been associated with an increased likelihood of "trading sex," or exchanging sexual favors for money, drugs, shelter, food, or other necessities (Burnette et al., 2008; Farley, 2004).

The association between trading sex and sexual victimization—particularly childhood sexual trauma—has been documented by several large-scale investigations of women in the civilian population. For example, among a large cross-sectional sample of women (n = 3,346) enrolled in a multisite HIV prevention trial, those who reported a history of childhood sexual trauma were twice as likely than those who did not report this history to have ever traded sex for money or drugs (NIMH [National Institute of Mental Health] Multisite HIV Prevention Trial Group, 2001). A similar pattern of findings (i.e., a nearly fourfold increased likelihood of trading sex for those with a history of childhood sexual abuse vs. non-maltreated controls) was observed among 426 women who participated in a 30-year prospective study of the effects of child abuse (Wilson & Widom, 2008). Relatedly, Noll, Trickett, and Putman (2003) documented a prospective relationship between childhood sexual abuse, subsequent rape or sexual assault in adolescence or adulthood, and high-risk sexual behaviors, including early sexual promiscuity and inconsistent use of birth control (see Seen, Carey, & Vanable, 2008, for a recent review of associations between childhood sexual abuse and risky sexual behaviors). High rates of trading sex have also been documented among incarcerated women (Hutton et al., 2001) and women with substance use disorders, including use of crack, cocaine, and injection drugs (Burnette et al., 2008; Edwards, Halpern, & Wechsberg, 2006; Logan, Cole, & Leukefeld, 2003).

Compared to women in the general population, women veterans experience disproportionately high rates of sexual violence across the lifespan as well as a high incidence of psychiatric illness (Fontana & Rosenheck, 1998; Fontana, Schwartz, & Rosenheck, 1997; Grossman et al., 1997; Pereira, 2002; Sadler, Booth, Cook, & Doebbeling, 2003; Sadler, Booth, Cook, Torner, & Doebbeling, 2001; Weitlauf et al., 2008). For these women, sexual trauma also may include military sexual trauma (MST), or the experience of sexual assault and/or harassment during one's military tour of duty. Approximately 22% of women veterans screened by the Department of Veteran Affairs (VA) are positive for MST compared to 1% of men (Kimerling, Gima, Smith, Street, & Frayne, 2007).

Previous investigators have posited that characteristics of the military setting and culture may exacerbate the negative consequences of MST as compared to sexual violence that occurs in civilian arenas (Kimerling et al., 2007). For example, MST generally occurs in the setting in which the victim lives and works, and close proximity to the perpetrator may increase feelings of helpless and risk for revictimization (National Center for Posttraumatic Stress Disorder & Department of Veteran Affairs, 2004). The strong organizational cohesion fostered within military units may result in conditions that interfere with victims' willingness or ability to report their experience of sexual violence and receive appropriate care (Kilpatrick, 1983). Thus, unique aspects of sexual violence that occurs within the military may compromise victims' posttrauma adjustment and contribute to long-term risks for adverse mental and physical health effects. Consistent with this perspective, MST is associated with a greater likelihood of developing PTSD than either childhood sexual abuse or civilian sexual assault (Suris, Lind, Kashner, Borman, & Petty, 2004).

To date, no empirical investigation has examined associations between trading sex and the experience of sexual violence that occurs during the course of military service. As a first step toward addressing this gap in the literature, the current study examined associations between MST and trading sex among women veterans consecutively recruited from a VA outpatient mental health clinic to participate in an HIV risk study. We hypothesized that compared to women without a history of MST, those with MST would report higher lifetime rates of trading sex. Another aim was to examine whether MST confers a unique risk for trading sex above the effects of other variables known to be associated with this risky sexual behavior. These other variables included substance use and childhood sexual trauma, both of which have been associated with trading sex in civilian samples.

METHODS

Participants

Participants were enrolled in a cross-sectional study of HIV risks and seroprevalence rates among women veterans receiving outpatient mental health care at the Durham VA Medical Center's Comprehensive Women's Health Center between 2001 and 2003. Consecutive patients who met eligibility criteria (i.e., patients were identified chronologically, in the order they presented for treatment at this clinic) were provided information about the study and procedures and were offered an opportunity to participate. Eligibility criteria included being age 18 or older; being fluent in English; and meeting criteria for a serious mental illness, defined as major depressive disorder, schizophrenia, schizoaffective disorder, bipolar I disorder, or PTSD as diagnosed by a detailed medical record review using a checklist to confirm *Diagnostic and Statistical Manual of Mental Disorders* (4th ed. [*DSM–IV*]) diagnostic criteria and a consensus review of the diagnosis by an attending psychiatrist (for the complete study methodology, see Rosenberg et al., 2003). A total of 34% of participants carried more than one of the Axis I diagnoses assessed for study eligibility (thus percentages sum to >100%): major depression = 76%, schizophrenia spectrum = 3%, bipolar I = 8%, PTSD = 48%.

Of 218 patients approached, 18 declined to participate and 200 were enrolled. Reasons provided for refusal to participate were as follows: afraid of blood tests (n = 2), anxious about study participation (n = 1), too busy (n = 5), not interested (n = 4), and not stated (n = 6). Assessment interviews were conducted prior to blood draws; no participant was found to be HIV positive. This study was approved by the Durham VA Medical Center's institutional review board, and all participants provided written informed consent.

Measures

Data were derived from two sources: medical record reviews and structured assessment interviews. Medical record reviews were conducted to determine diagnoses, as described above, and history of MST. The 1-hr assessment interview was composed of standardized measures, described below, that included sociodemographic characteristics, exposure to childhood sexual trauma, current substance use disorder, and sexual risk behaviors. Assessments were conducted in private offices by two trained interviewers who were experienced with this patient population.

Substance use disorders. Current alcohol and drug use disorders were assessed with the 18-item Dartmouth Assessment of Lifestyle Instrument (DALI; Rosenberg et al., 1998), a validated screening measure of current alcohol, cannabis, or cocaine abuse or dependence, which subsume the most commonly diagnosed substance use disorders among psychiatric patients. The DALI was specifically developed and validated for use with persons with mental illness, and it has demonstrated strong test–retest reliability and classification accuracy among persons with mental illness (Rosenberg et al., 1998). Current substance use disorder was coded for any participant who screened positive on this instrument for current alcohol, cannabis, or cocaine abuse or dependence.

MST. Mandatory MST screening of all VA users is conducted through a clinical reminder in the VA electronic medical record. This brief screening tool asks, "While you were in the military: A) Did you receive uninvited and unwanted sexual attention, such as touching, cornering, pressure for sexual favors, or verbal remarks? B) Did someone ever use force or threat of force to have sexual contact with you against your will?" Validated against clinical interviews using established assessment instruments, Question A has a sensitivity of .92 and a specificity of .89; Question B has a sensitivity of .89 and a specificity of .90 (Kimerling et al., 2007). Although specific item responses are not provided, positive MST screens (indicating an affirmative response to at least one of the two screening questions) are flagged in the electronic medical record. As an experience of MST is sometimes revealed subsequent to the completion of the clinical reminder, MST status was determined on the basis of these screening results as well as a review of chart notes. In 14 cases (7%), the review of chart notes indicated that a patient who had screened negative for MST on the mandatory clinical reminder later reported a history of MST to a provider (e.g., in the course of psychotherapy). In these cases, the patient was coded positive for MST for study analyses.

Childhood sexual abuse. The Sexual Abuse Exposure Questionnaire (SAEQ) was used to screen for the experience of sexual trauma before age 16 (Rodriguez, Ryan, Vande Kemp, & Foy, 1997; Ryan, Rodriguez, Rowan, & Foy, 1992). The SAEQ asks respondents whether they experienced any of 10 unwanted sexual experiences before age 16, ranging from being flashed to having sexual intercourse. A factor analysis of data from 1,000 respondents yielded a single factor reflecting unwanted sexual experiences, and test–retest reliability coefficients for SAEQ items have ranged from .73 to .94 (Rodriguez et al., 1997; Ryan et al., 1992). The composite variable any childhood sexual trauma was coded dichotomously and reflected an affirmative response to any of the 10 SAEQ items. Three additional dichotomous variables were created to reflect the type of childhood sexual trauma: non-contact, contact without penetration, and contact with penetration.

Trading sex. A composite variable, trading sex, was coded for affirmative responses to either of the following two questions from the AIDS Risk Inventory (ARI; Chawarski, Pakes, & Schottenfeld, 1998): "In your lifetime, have you ever had unprotected sex in exchange for money, food, a place to stay, or other things, even once?" and "In your lifetime, have you ever had unprotected sex in exchange for drugs (any kind), even once?" The ARI was developed to assess risk of HIV infection by querying about risk behaviors associated with drug use and sexual practices and by assessing knowledge of HIV prevention. In persons with mental illness, the ARI is able to discriminate between high- and low-risk HIV behaviors and to reliably assess risky behavior patterns (Chawarski et al., 1998).

Analyses

Means and percentages were computed to describe patient demographic, clinical, and behavioral characteristics for the total sample and by MST status. The bivariate relationship between each patient characteristic and MST status was analyzed using Wald chi-square statistics.

The bivariate relationship between trading sex and MST status, as well as bivariate relationships between trading sex and sociodemographic characteristics, current substance use disorder, and childhood sexual trauma history, were analyzed using unadjusted logistic regression models. Variables selected a priori for the adjusted trading sex logistic model included MST, substance use, and childhood sexual trauma. Sociodemographic characteristics that were statistically significant in bivariate analyses with trading sex were also included in this model. In addition, the any childhood sexual trauma variable was selected for inclusion in the multivariable model in lieu of the subtypes of childhood sexual trauma.

All analyses were conducted using SAS 9.2. (SAS Institute, Cary, NC); a p value of .05 (two-tailed) was used to assign significance for all statistical tests. Analyzed variables had minimal amounts of missing data; percentages reported in text and tables exclude participants with missing data.

RESULTS

Sample characteristics are presented in Table 1. The average age of the respondents was 45.5 years; 47% were ethnic minorities (87.2% of whom were African American). All had at least a high school education, and 90% had obtained some education beyond high school. Relatively few (14.5%) had ever served in a combat zone. A current substance use disorder (i.e., a positive screen on the DALI for current alcohol, cannabis, or cocaine abuse or dependence) was noted for 11.5% of participants. The rate of any childhood sexual trauma was high: 68.5% of participants endorsed at least one sexual trauma item on the SAEQ, 55% endorsed exposure to non-contact events, and 59% had been exposed to events that had included some contact but no physical penetration. More severe forms of childhood sexual abuse involving penetration were reported by 30.5% of the sample.

TABLE 1 Bivariate Associations of Patient Variables with MST Status

Variable	Total (N = 200)	MST (n = 134)	No MST (n = 66)	OR	95% CI
Sociodemographics					
Age, *M* (*SD*)	45.5 (7.9)	45.4 (7.6)	45.7 (8.6)	0.995	[0.96, 1.03]
Ethnic minority	94 (47.0)	60 (44.8)	34 (51.5)	0.76	[0.42, 1.38]
Education beyond high school	180 (90.0)	119 (88.8)	61 (92.4)	0.65	[0.23, 1.88]
Lives in own house/apartment	166 (83.0)	107 (79.9)	59 (89.4)	0.47	[0.19, 1.15]
Currently employed	70 (35.0)	40 (29.9)	30 (45.5)	0.51*	[0.28, 0.94]
Currently married	71 (35.5)	40 (29.9)	31 (47.0)	0.48	[0.28, 0.94]
Served in combat zone	29 (14.5)	18 (13.4)	11 (16.7)	0.78	[0.26, 0.88]
Current substance use disorder	23 (11.5)	19 (14.2)	4 (6.1)	2.56	[0.83, 7.86]
Any childhood sexual trauma	137 (68.5)	102 (76.1)	35 (53.0)	2.82**	[1.51, 5.28]
Non-contact sexual trauma	110 (55.0)	85 (63.4)	25 (37.9)	2.85***	[1.55, 5.23]
Flash/expose sexual parts	95 (47.5)	73 (54.5)	22 (33.3)		
Watch dress/use bathroom	44 (22.2)	39 (29.5)	5 (7.6)		
Make watch sexual acts	29 (14.6)	27 (20.3)	2 (3.0)		
Make pose for sexy pictures	4 (2.1)	4 (3.1)	0 (0.0)		
Contact without penetration	118 (59.0)	93 (69.4)	25 (37.9)	3.72***	[2.00, 6.90]
Private parts touched	115 (57.8)	90 (67.7)	25 (37.9)		
Make touch another	68 (34.5)	56 (42.4)	12 (19.5)		
Make perform oral sex	28 (14.2)	25 (19.1)	3 (4.5)		
Perform oral sex on you	22 (11.4)	20 (15.7)	2 (3.0)		
Contact with penetration	60 (30.5)	49 (37.4)	11 (16.7)	2.99**	[1.43, 6.25]
Make have intercourse	60 (30.5)	49 (37.4)	11 (16.7)		
Make have anal sex[a]	11 (5.6)	10 (7.6)	1 (1.5)		

Notes. Data are n (%) except where noted. MST = military sexual trauma; OR = odds ratio; CI = confidence interval.

[a]All participants who reported being made to have anal sex also reported being made to have intercourse. Therefore, the overall contact with penetration variable and the made to have intercourse variable have the same analytic results.

*$p < .05$.

**$p < .01$.

***$p < .001$.

More than two thirds (67%) screened positive for MST. Compared to those without MST, a smaller proportion of those with MST were currently employed and currently married (see Table 1). Those with MST were otherwise demographically similar to those without MST. Compared to those without MST, those with MST were significantly more likely to report having experienced childhood sexual victimization as well as each subtype of childhood sexual trauma (i.e., non-contact, contact without penetration, and contact with penetration). Table 1 also presents frequencies and percentages, for the full sample and for the subsamples of those with and without MST, for each type of childhood sexual abuse queried on the SAEQ.

Table 2 documents the bivariate associations between patient variables and trading sex. Of the 200 women in the sample, 39 (19.7%) reported a lifetime history of trading sex. As hypothesized, those who reported trading

TABLE 2 Bivariate Associations of Patient Variables with Lifetime History of Trading Sex

Variable	Traded sex ($N = 39$)	Did not trade sex ($N = 159$)	OR	95% CI
Sociodemographics				
Age, *M* (*SD*)	45.2 (7.6)	45.7 (8.0)	0.99	[0.95, 1.04]
Ethnic minority	16 (41.0)	78 (49.1)	0.72	[0.36, 1.47]
Education beyond high school	30 (76.9)	148 (93.1)	0.25**	[0.09, 0.65]
Lives in own house/apartment	30 (76.9)	135 (84.9)	0.59	[0.25, 1.40]
Currently employed	18 (46.2)	50 (31.4)	1.87	[0.92, 3.81]
Currently married	15 (38.5)	55 (34.6)	1.18	[0.57, 2.44]
Served in combat zone	2 (5.1)	27 (17.0)	0.26	[0.06, 1.16]
Current substance use disorder	9 (23.1)	14 (8.8)	3.11*	[1.23, 7.84]
MST	34 (87.2)	100 (62.9)	4.01**	[1.49, 10.82]
Childhood sexual trauma				
Any childhood sexual trauma	33 (84.6)	103 (64.8)	2.99*	[1.18, 7.57]
Non-contact	27 (69.2)	82 (51.6)	2.11*	[1.00, 4.46]
Contact without penetration	31 (79.5)	86 (54.1)	3.29**	[1.42, 7.60]
Contact with penetration	15 (38.5)	45 (28.8)	1.54	[0.74, 3.21]

Notes. Data are *n* (%) except where noted. OR = odds ratio; CI = confidence interval; MST = military sexual trauma.
$^{*}p < .05$.
$^{**}p < .01$.

sex had a higher rate of MST than those who did not report a history of trading sex (see Table 2). Trading sex was also significantly associated with less educational achievement, higher rates of childhood sexual trauma, and a greater likelihood of current substance use disorders.

Multivariable logistic regression was used to examine the adjusted association between MST and trading sex with current substance use, any childhood sexual trauma, and education as covariates. Results of the adjusted trading sex logistic regression model are presented in Table 3. Those with MST had a higher odds of reporting trading sex than those without MST: odds ratio = 3.26, $p = .025$, 95% confidence interval = [1.16, 9.18]. The c-statistic for the adjusted logistic regression model was 0.74.

TABLE 3 Adjusted Logistic Regression Analysis of Education, Substance Use, Childhood Sexual Trauma, and MST Status in Relation to Trading Sex

Variable	OR	95% CI
Education beyond high school	0.28*	[0.10, 0.77]
Current substance use disorder	2.35	[0.87, 6.31]
Any childhood sexual trauma	2.46	[0.93, 6.53]
MST	3.26*	[1.16, 9.18]

Notes. MST = military sexual trauma; OR = odds ratio; CI = confidence interval.
$^{*}p < .05$.

DISCUSSION

To our knowledge, the current study is among the first to investigate the risky practice of trading sex among women veterans. Among 200 women enrolled for treatment at a VA outpatient mental health clinic, nearly 1 in 5 reported a lifetime history of trading sex. As predicted, a history of MST was significantly and independently associated with trading sex, even after we adjusted for the effects of current substance use disorder, childhood sexual trauma, and education (education was also significant in adjusted analyses).

As would be anticipated in a cohort seeking mental health services, the rate of MST in the current sample (67%) was higher than the reported prevalence rate of 22% among the general population of women VA clinic users (Kimerling et al., 2007). Rates of substance use disorders and childhood sexual trauma observed in this sample were also higher than those reported for the general population of women veterans (Sadler et al., 2003; Stern et al., 2000) but still within the range of previous reports of treatment-seeking women veterans (Butterfield, McIntyre, Stechuchak, Nanda, & Bastian, 1998; Fontana & Rosenheck, 1998). Also as anticipated, and consistent with previous findings, MST was associated with high rates of childhood sexual trauma (Merrill et al., 1999; Sadler et al., 2003; Suris et al., 2004): Those with MST were more likely to have experienced all three subtypes of childhood sexual abuse (non-contact, contact without penetration, and contact with penetration).

In this help-seeking sample, nearly 20% reported a lifetime history of trading sex, and among the subgroup of those with MST, 25% reported trading sex versus 8% of those without MST. To place this finding in context, we should note that the rate of trading sex observed for those with MST in the current study is somewhat lower than rates previously reported for several other cohorts documented to be at increased risk for trading sex, which have ranged from 30% for female prisoners (Hutten et al., 2001) to 44%–51% among help-seeking women with substance use disorders (Burnette et al., 2008; Edwards et al., 2006). However, the 25% lifetime prevalence of trading sex for those with MST is well within the range reported for some at-risk cohorts, including 10%–28% of homeless and runaway youths (Greene, Ennett, & Ringwalt, 1999); 13%–17% of female survivors of childhood physical abuse, sexual abuse, or neglect (Wilson & Widom, 2008); and 12%–21% of women recruited from sexually transmitted disease clinics and health service organizations (Hutton, Lyketsos, Zenilman, Thompson, & Erbelding, 2004; NIMH Multisite HIV Prevention Trial Group, 2001). In contrast, Wilson and Widom (2008) reported that only 4% of female non-maltreated controls acknowledged ever trading sex.

MST was significantly and independently associated with trading sex in the adjusted analyses. These findings extend previously observed associations between a history of sexual trauma and trading sex in civilian female cohorts (Edwards et al., 2006; Farley & Barkan, 1998; Hutton et al., 2001; Miner, Flitter, & Robinson, 2006; NIMH Multisite HIV Prevention Trial Group, 2001; Noll, Horowitz, Bonanno, Trickett, & Putnam, 2003; Noll, Trickett, et al., 2003; Widom & Kuhns, 1996; Wilson & Widom, 2008). These results are also consistent with prior empirical and clinical evidence that suggests that MST is associated with more negative outcomes than civilian sexual trauma (e.g., Kimerling et al., 2007; Suris et al., 2004). When considered in the context of prevalence rates reported for other at-risk groups, the current findings suggest that help-seeking women with MST may be considered at relatively high risk for engaging in trading sex. As causal pathways and temporal associations cannot be inferred from cross-sectional data, more work is needed to examine the nature of these relationships. However, the present findings are consistent with reports of prior investigations and underscore the pernicious influence of sexual victimization across the lifespan. These findings thus serve both to extend understanding of the link between sexual violence and sex trading and to deepen awareness of the potentially severe consequences associated with MST exposure in female veterans.

The extant literature shows all too well that trading sex is associated with significant threats to physical and emotional well-being, including, to name a few, heightened risk of sexual and physical violence, physical injury, PTSD, depression, substance abuse, traumatic brain injury, poverty, sexually transmitted diseases, HIV/AIDS, cervical cancer, suicide, and murder (Farley, 2004). This literature also indicates that the longer one engages in trading sex, the greater the risk of these adverse outcomes. On the basis of the current findings, we posit that the prevalence of trading sex is an underdetected aspect of the often complex clinical picture for some women veterans, in particular those who have experienced MST.

Although preliminary, these findings yield several important implications for clinical practice and future research. Clinically speaking, there is a need for thorough and sensitive assessment, early intervention, and preventive efforts. Potential early interventions could include routine education and skills training around sexually transmitted disease transmission and substance abuse issues, including relapse prevention and assistance seeking employment, benefits, and stable housing. Preventive intervention efforts may target social issues related to trading sex, particularly among women veterans with histories of child sexual abuse, MST, and substance use disorders. In view of the further association of lower education and trading sex, prevention efforts also may include consideration of health literacy. Further research that explores the prevalence, consequences, and treatment needs of these women is warranted and should more fully evaluate factors associated with the experience of MST that may augment vulnerability to sex trade.

As with all studies, the current investigation has several limitations. The sample was limited to a convenience sample enrolled in a cross-sectional study of HIV risks and seroprevalence rates among women veterans with a serious mental illness receiving outpatient mental health care at a VA medical center. Only 18 (8.3%) out of 218 women approached declined to participate (see the stated reasons in "Participants"). Still, the results may not generalize to other populations. Diagnoses, which included major depressive disorder, schizophrenia, schizoaffective disorder, bipolar I disorder, and PTSD, were based on chart diagnoses and record review to ensure that *DSM–IV* criteria were met, as opposed to structured clinical interviews. Our measure of current substance use was the DALI, a brief screening instrument that assesses alcohol, cannabis, and cocaine abuse and dependence, which represent the most frequently diagnosed substance use disorders among psychiatric populations. Thus, less common types of substance use (e.g., amphetamine use, inhalant use) would not have been detected. Although we recruited an ethnically diverse sample, which may be considered a strength of this study that enhances its generalizability, data were not available to fully capitalize on potentially influential elements underlying the construct of ethnic diversity (e.g., acculturation, cultural values). Also, the current study only examined the lifetime occurrence of unprotected sex in exchange for money, drugs, shelter, food, or other things. We did not assess the frequency of this behavior or the number of partners, which have been shown to be associated with health outcomes such as HIV infection (Astemborski, Vlahov, Warren, Solomon, & Nelson, 1994). Likewise, the frequency of childhood sexual abuse or MST, or the time since victimization, was not assessed, nor were we able to assess adult sexual trauma that occurred outside the window of military service. Finally, given the sensitive nature of the content covered by the assessment interview, social desirability concerns may have limited participants' willingness to disclose socially stigmatizing behaviors and experiences to study staff (Catania, Gibson, Chitwood, & Coates, 1990), particularly in the context of a blood test for HIV/AIDS. Although no participant was found to be HIV positive, anticipation of the venipuncture that occurred after the assessment interviews could have been a significant source of anxiety (either because of the potentially stigmatizing effects of a positive result or because venipuncture can be anxiety producing more generally) and thus could have impacted participants' responses to the interview questions. To minimize social desirability concerns and participant anxiety, all interviewers had previous experience with similar cohorts and were extensively trained to administer the structured assessment interview.

Despite these limitations, this is the first report of the association between MST and the particularly dangerous sexual risk behavior of trading sex. The results extend previous findings of adverse mental health and functional outcomes among women veterans with MST (Butterfield et al., 1998; Suris, Lind, Kashner, & Borman, 2007; Yaeger, Himmelfarb, Cammack, & Mintz, 2006). MST plays a prominent role in women veteran's histories of sexual victimization and thus may merit increased and more targeted screening and prevention to mitigate against risk behaviors, such as trading sex, and intervention efforts to address associated consequences and subsequent risks among those who have engaged in this behavior.

REFERENCES

Astemborski, J., Vlahov, D., Warren, D., Solomon, L., & Nelson, K. E. (1994). The trading of sex for drugs or money and HIV seropositivity among female intravenous drug users. *American Journal of Public Health, 84*, 382–387.

Burnette, M. L., Lucas, E., Ilgen, M., Frayne, S. M., Mayo, J., & Weitlauf, J. C. (2008). Prevalence and health correlates of prostitution among patients entering treatment for substance use disorders. *Archives of General Psychiatry, 65*, 337–344.

Butterfield, M. I., McIntyre, L. M., Stechuchak, K. M., Nanda, K., & Bastian, L. A. (1998). Mental disorder symptoms in veteran women: Impact of physical and sexual assault. *Journal of American Medical Women Association, 53*(4), 198–200.

Catania, J. A., Gibson, D., Chitwood, D., & Coates, T. (1990). Methodological problems in AIDS behavioral research: Influences of measurement error and participation bias in studies of sexual behavior. *Psychological Bulletin, 108*, 339–362.

Chawarski, M. C., Pakes, J., & Schottenfeld, R. S. (1998). Assessment of HIV risk. *Journal of Addictive Disorders, 17*, 49–59.

Dobie, D. J., Kivlahan, D. R., Maynard, C., Bush, K. R., Davis, T. M., & Bradley, K. A. (2004). Posttraumatic stress disorder in female veterans: Association with self-reported health problems and functional impairment. *Archives of Internal Medicine, 164*, 394–400.

Edwards, J. M., Halpern, C. T., & Wechsberg, W. M. (2006). Correlates of exchanging sex for drugs or money among women who use crack cocaine. *AIDS Education and Prevention, 18*, 420–429.

Farley, M. (2004). "Bad for the body, bad for the heart": Prostitution harms women even if legalized or decriminalized. *Violence Against Women, 10*, 1087–1125.

Farley, M., & Barkan, H. (1998). Prostitution, violence, and posttraumatic stress disorder. *Women's Health, 27*(3), 37–49.

Fontana, A., & Rosenheck, R. (1998). Duty-related and sexual stress in the etiology of PTSD among women veterans who seek treatment. *Psychiatric Services, 49*, 658–662.

Fontana, A., Schwartz, L. S., & Rosenheck, R. (1997). Posttraumatic stress disorder among female Vietnam veterans: A causal model of etiology. *American Journal of Public Health, 87*, 169–175.

Frayne, S. M., Skinner, K. M., Sullivan, L. M., & Freund, K. M. (2003). Sexual assault while in the military: Violence as a predictor of cardiac risk? *Violence and Victims, 18*, 219–225.

Greene, J. M., Ennett, S. T., & Ringwalt, C. L. (1999). Prevalence and correlates of survival sex among runaway and homeless youth. *American Journal of Public Health, 89*, 1406–1409.

Grossman, L. S., Willer, J. K., Stovall, J. G., McRae, S. G., Maxwell, S., & Nelson, R. (1997). Underdiagnosis of PTSD and substance use disorders in hospitalized female veterans. *Psychiatric Services*, *48*, 393–395.

Hutton, H. E., Lyketsos, C. G., Zenilman, J. M., Thompson, R. E., & Erbelding, E. J. (2004). Depression and HIV risk behaviors among patients in a sexually transmitted disease clinic. *American Journal of Psychiatry*, *161*, 912–914.

Hutton, H. E., Treisman, G. J., Hunt, W. R., Fishman, M., Kendig, N., Swetz, A., & Lyketsos, C. G. (2001). HIV risk behaviors and their relationship to post-traumatic stress disorder among women prisoners. *Psychiatric Services*, *52*, 508–513.

Kilpatrick, D. G. (1983). Rape victims: Detection, assessment and treatment. *The Clinical Psychologist*, *36*, 92–95.

Kimerling, R., Gima, K., Smith, M. W., Street, A., & Frayne, S. (2007). The Veterans Health Administration and military sexual trauma. *American Journal of Public Health*, *97*, 1–7.

Letourneau, E. J., Holmes, M., & Chasedunn-Roark, J. (1999). Gynecologic health consequences to victims of interpersonal violence. *Women's Health Issues*, *9*, 115–120.

Logan, T. K., Cole, J., & Leukefeld, C. (2003). Gender differences in the context of sex exchange among individuals with a history of crack use. *Education and Prevention*, *15*, 448–464.

Merrill, L. L., Newell, C. E., Thomsen, C. J., Gold, S. R., Milner, J. S., Koss, M. P., & Rosswork, S. G. (1999). Childhood abuse and sexual revictimization in a female Navy recruit sample. *Journal of Traumatic Stress*, *12*(2), 211–225.

Miner, M. H., Flitter, J. M., & Robinson, B. B. E. (2006). Association of sexual revictimization with sexuality and psychological function. *Journal of Interpersonal Violence*, *21*, 503–524.

National Center for Post-Traumatic Stress Disorder & Department of Veteran Affairs. (2004). *Iraq War clinician guide* (2nd ed.). Retrieved from http://www.ptsd.va.gov/professional/manuals/iraq-war-clinician-guide.asp

NIMH Multisite HIV Prevention Trial Group. (2001). A test of factors mediating the relationship between unwanted sexual activity during childhood and risky sexual practices among women enrolled in the NIMH Multisite HIV Prevention Trial. *Women's Work, Health and Quality of Life*, *33*(1–2), 163–180.

Noll, J. G., Horowitz, L. A., Bonanno, G. A., Trickett, P. K., & Putnam, F. W. (2003). Revictimization and self-harm in females who experienced childhood sexual abuse: Results from a prospective study. *Journal of Interpersonal Violence*, *18*, 1452–1471.

Noll, J. G., Trickett, P. K., & Putnam, F. W. (2003). A prospective investigation of the impact of childhood sexual abuse on the development of sexuality. *Journal of Consulting and Clinical Psychology*, *71*, 575–586.

Pereira, A. (2002). Combat trauma and the diagnosis of posttraumatic stress disorder in female and male veterans. *Military Medicine*, *167*, 23–27.

Reynolds, M. W., Peipert, J. F., Collins, B. (2000). Epidemiological issues of sexually transmitted diseases in sexual assault victims. *Obstetrical & Gynecological Survey*, *55*, 51–57.

Rodriguez, N., Ryan, S. W., Vande Kemp, H., & Foy, D. W. (1997). Posttraumatic stress disorder in adult female survivors of childhood sexual abuse: A comparison study. *Journal of Consulting and Clinical Psychology*, *65*, 53–59.

Rosenberg, S. D., Drake, R. E., Wolford, G. L., Mueser, K. T., Oxman, T. E., Vidaver, R. M., . . . Luckoor, R. (1998). Dartmouth Assessment of Lifestyle Instrument (DALI): A substance use disorder screen for people with severe mental illness. *American Journal of Psychiatry*, *155*, 232–238.

Rosenberg, S. D., Swanson, J. W., Wolford, G. L., Osher, F. C., Swartz, M. S., Essock, S. M., . . . the Five-Site Health and Risk Study Research Team. (2003). The five-site health and risk study of blood-borne infections among persons with severe mental illness. *Psychiatric Services*, *54*, 827–835.

Ryan, S. W., Rodriguez, N., Rowan, A., & Foy, D. W. (1992, August). *Psychometric analysis of the Sexual Abuse Exposure Questionnaire (SAEQ)*. Paper presented at the Annual Meeting of the American Psychological Association, Washington, DC.

Sadler, A. G., Booth, B. M., Cook, B. L., & Doebbeling, B. N. (2003). Factors associated with women's risk of rape in the military environment. *American Journal of Industrial Medicine*, *43*(3), 262–273.

Sadler, A. G., Booth, B. M., Cook, B. L., Torner, J. C., & Doebbeling, B. N. (2001). The military environment: Risk factors for women's non-fatal assaults. *Journal of Occupational and Environmental Medicine*, *43*, 325–334.

Seen, T. E., Carey, M. P., & Vanable, P. A. (2008). Childhood and adolescent sexual abuse and subsequent sexual risk behavior: Evidence from controlled studies, methodological critique, and suggestions for research. *Clinical Psychology Review*, *28*, 711–735.

Stern, A., Wolfe, J., Daley, J., Zaslavsky, A., Roper, S. F., & Wilson, K. (2000). Changing demographic characteristics of women veterans: Results from a national sample. *Military Medicine*, *165*, 773–780.

Suris, A., & Lind, L. (2008). Military sexual trauma: A review of prevalence and associated health consequences in veterans. *Trauma, Violence, & Abuse*, *9*(4), 250–269.

Suris, A., Lind, L., Kashner, M., & Borman, P. D. (2007). Mental health, quality of life, and health functioning in women veterans: Differential outcomes associated with military and civilian sexual assault. *Journal of Interpersonal Violence*, *22*, 179–196.

Suris, A., Lind, L., Kashner, T. M., Borman, P. D., & Petty, F. (2004). Sexual assault in women veterans: An examination of PTSD risk, health care utilization, and cost of care. *Psychosomatic Medicine*, *66*, 749–756.

Weitlauf, J. C., Finney, J. W., Ruzek, J. I., Lee, T. T., Thrailkill, A., Jones, S., & Frayne, S. (2008). Distress and pain during pelvic examinations: Effect of sexual violence. *Obstetrics and Gynecology*, *112*, 1343–1350.

Widom, C. S., & Kuhns, J. B. (1996). Childhood victimization and subsequent risk for promiscuity, prostitution, and teenage pregnancy: A prospective study. *American Journal of Public Health*, *86*, 1607–1612.

Wilson, H. W., & Widom, C. S. (2008). An examination of risky sexual behavior and HIV in victims of child abuse and neglect: A 30-year follow-up. *Health Psychology*, *27*(2), 149–158.

Yaeger, D., Himmelfarb, N., Cammack, A., & Mintz, J. (2006). *DSM-IV* diagnosed posttraumatic stress disorder in women veterans with and without military sexual trauma. *Journal of General Internal Medicine*, *21*(Suppl. 3), S65–S69.

Reengineering Gender Relations in Modern Militaries: An Evolutionary Perspective

REBECCA J. HANNAGAN, PhD

Department of Political Science, Northern Illinois University, DeKalb, Illinois, USA

HOLLY ARROW, PhD

Department of Psychology & Institute of Cognitive and Decision Sciences, University of Oregon, Eugene, Oregon, USA

This article presents an evolutionary framework for understanding the sexual assault of women in the military. We specify the evolutionary underpinnings of tensions among heterosexual males, among heterosexual females, and between males and females and discuss how these tensions have played out in the strongly gendered context of warrior culture. In the absence of cultural interventions that take into account deep-seated conceptions of women in the military as unwelcome intruders, sexual resources for military men, or both, military women operate in an environment in which sexual assault may be deployed to enact and defend traditional military structures. We discuss how unit norms are likely to affect the choice of strategies by men and by women and how the resulting behaviors—including celibacy, consensual sex, and sexual assault—should affect horizontal and vertical unit cohesion. The framework is intended to guide future data collection in theoretically coherent ways and to inform the framing and enforcement of policies regarding both consensual and non-consensual sex among military personnel.

The authors thank John Orbell for his many valuable contributions to launching this project; 1Lt Andrea Wolfe for input on Air Force policies and practices; the Institute of Cognitive and Decision Sciences for hosting the Evolutionary Perspectives on War Conference in October 2008, where the authors conceived this project; and Dropbox and Skype for providing essential long-distance collaboration tools.

Recent studies suggest that a substantial proportion of military women (and a smaller proportion of military men) experience sexual harassment, coercion, and assault during their service (Friedman, 2006; Sadler, Booth, Cook, & Doebbeling, 2003; Yaeger, Himmelfarb, Cammack, & Mintz, 2006). Military sexual assault (MSA) contributes to the incidence of posttraumatic stress disorder (PTSD) in veterans. Among Gulf War veterans, being sexually assaulted increased the odds of developing PTSD to a greater degree than did combat experience for both men and women (Kang, Dalager, Mahan, & Ishii, 2005). Of the 2 million Americans who have served in Iraq and Afghanistan since 2001, 11% (more than 220,000) have been women (Alvarez, 2009). If estimated prevalence rates for female veterans from the Vietnam and post-Vietnam eras (Sadler et al., 2003) are comparable for this population, between a quarter and a third of these women have experienced one or more completed or attempted rapes.

As mandated by Congress, steps have been taken to assess the problem of MSA in the U.S. military. Systematic, reliable data on MSA within the armed forces are not yet available, however. Reporting in December 2009, the Defense Task Force on Sexual Assault in the Military Services found the Department of Defense procedures for collecting data about MSA to be "lacking in accuracy, reliability, and validity" (Iasiello et al., 2009, p. 77). Other sources of data include responses to universal screening questions by the Veterans Health Administration (e.g., Kimerling, Gima, Smith, Street, & Frayne, 2007), clinical interviews of veterans receiving treatment (e.g., Yaeger et al., 2006), and self-report responses to surveys and questionnaires (e.g., Murdoch, Polusny, Hodges, & O'Brien, 2004). The variance in reported prevalence rates of MSA among women, from less than 5% to more than 70% (for a review of the studies, see Suris & Lind, 2008), suggests that all estimates should be treated with caution. Data on the men (studies typically find that close to 100% of perpetrators are male) who are assaulting military women (and, less commonly, other men) are even sparser, and studies (e.g., Sadler et al., 2003) that collect data on characteristics of both victims and their assailants are exceedingly rare.

Theoretical accounts of MSA are also in an early state of development. New theorizing about wartime rape (Henry, Ward, & Hirshberg, 2004; Littlewood, 1997; Stiglmayer, 1994) was prompted by widespread sexual violence during the Rwanda genocide and Balkan conflicts. However, these accounts focus on the rape of civilians officially defined as the enemy. MSA generally occurs among members of the same military. Models of sexual harassment in the civilian workplace have also been applied to the military (e.g., Fitzgerald, Drasgow, & Magley, 1999). However, it appears that the direct antecedents of sexual harassment (job gender context and organizational tolerance) are only indirectly associated with sexual assault in the same context (Harned, Ormerod, Palmieri, Collinsworth, & Reed, 2002).

In this article, we offer a theoretical account of male-on-female MSA that integrates military culture and gender dynamics, guided by evolutionary theory. It does not cover the topic fully. In particular, the evolutionary grounding for our model offers little traction for explaining male-on-male sexual assault or the much rarer phenomenon of female assailants. Despite these limitations, we believe it can serve as a useful building block in developing a more comprehensive account of MSA to guide both research and practical efforts at reform.

We begin by specifying the evolutionary underpinnings of tensions among heterosexual males, among heterosexual females, and between males and females and then discuss how these tensions have played out in the strongly gendered context of warrior culture. As Goldstein (2001, p. 7) documented in his comprehensive study of gender and war, the strongest gender roles are those connected most closely with war. In this strongly gendered context, women in the military have frequently been viewed not as fellow soldiers but either as intruders or as a sexual resource to be exploited (Goldstein, 2001; Rosen, Knudson, & Fancher, 2003). In the absence of cultural interventions that take into account these deep-seated and long-standing conceptions, military women operate in an environment in which sexual assault may be deployed to defend traditional military structures.

THE EVOLUTIONARY LOGIC OF GENDERED RELATIONS

Gottschall (2004, p. 129) identified four theoretical frameworks that offer explanations for wartime rape: feminist theory, cultural pathology theory, strategic rape theory, and biosocial theory. The biosocial theory of wartime rape integrates sociocultural factors with the evolved sexual psychology of human males. Our approach is similar, although we pay attention to the evolved sexual psychology of females as well and focus on men and women who are serving in the same military.[1] The primary sociocultural factors we integrate are socialization practices and cultural gender norms common to both warrior bands and large-scale militaries across history.

The evolutionary logic of differential parental investment has shaped sex differences in mating strategies between heterosexual men and women (Trivers, 1972, 1974). The demands of pregnancy, lactation, and childrearing mean that women reliably invest more in offspring than do men. The mother's investment is more critical for a child's survival, and the smaller investment by males makes their fecundity more variable than females'. Sexual strategies shaped by these differences yield both conflict and cooperation within and among men and women. Although they evolved based on differential demands regarding mating, reproduction, and parenting, the implications of these sexual strategies can be activated in domains (such as war fighting) that appear on the surface to have little to do with reproduction.

Male Competition and Cooperation

Heterosexual men compete with one another to gain access to women (Daly & Wilson, 1978; Van Vugt, De Cremer, & Janssen, 2007), and this status competition can disrupt group living. For men, risk taking that might enable higher status and more mating opportunities is frequently worth the gamble of interpersonal violence (Campbell, 2002, p. 100). When violence is between groups instead of individuals, the stakes are even higher: the reproductive success of both oneself and one's blood relatives.

War can have both disastrously bad and spectacularly positive effects on male reproductive success, depending on whether warriors are on the losing or winning side. For the vanquished, ancestral war had potentially genocidal effects either on a whole group or on the male lines of descent within a group (Keeley, 1997; LeBlanc, 1999, p. 716). For men in the victorious group, collective access to women in the defeated population offers opportunities to father more offspring. Military prowess can also result in higher status and hence better mating success within one's own population. A link between military and reproductive success has been documented among Yanomamo men: *Unokais*, who have killed one or more enemies, have more wives and children than non-*unokais* (Chagnon, 1988).

Warriors are unlikely to prevail in war if they cannot cooperate effectively, and hence war provides a potent stimulus for men on the same side to reduce interpersonal conflict. Sharing the collective rewards of victory helps reduce intragroup sexual competition among men. The transfer of status competition to the intergroup level helps promote within-group cooperation among men (Van Vugt et al., 2007), creating a mutually reinforcing positive feedback loop that in turn promotes military effectiveness (Shils & Janowitz, 1948).

A strong hierarchy, which is typical of modern militaries, reduces the propensity for lower ranked males to challenge higher ranked males. This facilitates vertical cohesion, the bonds between men and their leaders (Griffith, 1988). Horizontal group bonding among men of the same rank reduces the intensity and lethality of competition within cohorts by inducing them to view one another as brothers with a mutual interest in survival. Men more than women value groups that affirm a common identity that ties all of the men to the group (Seeley, Gardner, Pennington, & Gabriel, 2003).

Cultural practices that bond groups of men together, such as initiation rites, are widespread. A study of 60 societies found that the prevalence of warfare was the best predictor of the severity of such initiation rites (Sosis, Kress, & Boster, 2007). In contemporary militaries, basic training exerts intense stress on recruits to reinforce a strong collective identity. These bonds strengthen in combat, developing into the tactical cohesion that holds units together and maintains effectiveness under fire (Greenbaum, 1979; Marshall, 1947). In this way, the social engineering of male bonding both damps down intragroup fighting over women and promotes victory in war.

When military socialization is designed to forge men into male-bonded groups, women are commonly viewed as a threat to group cohesion. Cross-cultural studies have documented an extremely common cultural pattern in which women's influence on men's hunting and war is seen as harmful. Taboos against women using weapons associated with these male activities (Brightman, 1996) effectively exclude women from the ranks of warriors. If this view of women as harmful intruders is normative for a group, sexual assault of military women may be used to protect the male-bonded unit. Assault may include gang rape, which both punishes women who are violating gender norms and binds the men in a collective deviant act (Bourke, 2007, p. 376). When women serve in support roles that the men do not view as threatening the integrity of the group, however, they may instead be valued as members of the society that the (male) warriors are defending.

Female Competition and Cooperation

Women compete to mate with the "best" men to ensure healthy children and to secure resources. However, women are much more likely than men to choose indirect forms of aggression over physical violence, as physical injury can impede effective childrearing (Campbell, 2002; Geary, 1998; Hrdy, 2000). Women also differ in how they deploy their sexual assets to attract resources from men, and this creates conflict. Those who have or are seeking committed male–female pair bonds are at odds with sexually promiscuous women who might threaten the channeling of resources to their children (Campbell, 2002; Geary, 1998; Hrdy, 2000).

This conflict drives the dynamic that unites wives against mistresses and prostitutes, promoting female alliances against women who use a different sexual strategy. Pair-bonded women also benefit from cooperation to share childrearing tasks and protect collective resources their children need. They may also ally with other women to reduce male sexual coercion (Gowaty, 2003; Hrdy, 2000; Low, 2001; Smuts, 1992; Zihlman, 1981)

Cultural practices that bond sizeable groups of unrelated women together in symbolic sisterhood appear to be less common than those that bond together unrelated bands of brothers. Although women have long been involved in war (De Pauw, 1998; Enloe, 2000; Goldstein, 2001), participation as warriors in formally organized units has been the exception rather than the rule. Outside of the domestic sphere, in which the women are related by blood or marriage, female coalitions are rarely as powerful as those formed by males (Low, 2001).

Differences in behavior evoked by intergroup as opposed to interpersonal contexts are weaker among women (Wildschut, Pinter, Vevea, Insko, & Schopler, 2003), and intergroup competition in particular has less impact on women's propensity to cooperate than it does on men's (Van Vugt et al., 2007). The lower importance of common identity for women (Seeley et al., 2003) makes it a less potent route to horizontal cohesion. This may be why military women prefer working with men: 8% agreed with the statement "I prefer to work with female soldiers," 63% disagreed, and 29% were undecided (Rosen et al., 1996).

Competition and Cooperation Among Men and Women

Differences in parental investment fuels a fundamental conflict between the sexes (Trivers, 1972, 1974). Men tend to favor strategies that improve their access to and control of female sexuality, whereas women seek to maintain control of their own sexuality and reproduction and reduce male sexual coercion (Geary, 1998; Gowaty, 2003; Hrdy, 2000). From a biosocial perspective, this conflict is at the root of the dominance struggles that are a major focus of feminist theory and scholarship (Smuts, 1992). Both perspectives recognize that strong male alliances help maintain male dominance and neutralize the impact of female alliances, reducing female autonomy and choice (Low, 2001).

The sexual strategies of men and women can also mesh cooperatively when men and women join in committed pair bonds. Mothers and fathers have a shared incentive to cooperate in successful childrearing (Hrdy, 2009). Given that conflict between the sexes is a source of solidarity among men and among women, what impact do these cooperative heterosexual pair bonds have on cohesion among and between men and women? Existing data present a mixed picture consistent with the complexity of the interwoven incentives for competition and cooperation both within and between the sexes.

For example, although some scholars link a masculinist warrior identity with rape-conducive norms (e.g., Morris, 1996), it appears that in male-only units, cohesion-promoting hypermasculinity at the group level is also positively associated with support for spouses (Rosen et al., 2003). This positive relationship was not found in mixed-gender combat support units. The explanation may lie in the power of male–female pairings to disrupt alliances among males when these pair bonds are not clearly separated from the male-bonded unit. When male alliances are critical to a group's survival, allied males may view intimate pair bonds with females as a source of tension that divides a man's loyalties and threatens group cohesion (Low, 2001; Smuts, 1992). From the paired male's point of view, friendly relations between his mate and other males in a group may spark jealousy and suspicion. In this way male–female pair bonds can make horizontal group cohesion problematic for both partners if the partners are serving in the same unit.

Across many societies and time periods, women have been treated as spoils of war by warriors on the winning side (Keeley, 1997), and this can put unattached women who are not pair-bonded at risk. The link between military success and male reproductive success is also affirmed by civilian and military women who reward military prowess with sex and shame men who avoid military service (Goldstein, 2001). Organized military brothels as a resource for maintaining morale (Moon, 1997; Stiglmayer, 1994) also affirm the view of women as a sexual resource to which military men are entitled. Rather than (or in addition to) paying for sex, military men may pursue their unattached female colleagues. Some military women will reciprocate the attention by embracing the opportunities for promiscuity, which may include trading sex for favors and for privileged access to higher status men. Women who reject the attention may be assaulted.

Sexual assault promoted by the "women as spoils" view is more about sex and less about power than the "women as intruders" dynamic. Force is a means to an end rather than the primary goal. Officers who use rank to coerce subordinate women into unwanted sex are also enacting and validating this view of women as a sexual resource. The goal is not to drive the women away but to claim them as a perquisite of high rank.

A conception of military women as neither intruders nor a sexual resource for military men is the ungendered professionalism (Rosen et al., 2003) promoted by Morris (1996) as an alternative to the hypermasculinity of traditional military culture. Treating women as comrades-in-arms promotes a model of cooperation that downplays gender and should also discourage sexual assault. From an evolutionary perspective, the most promising analogue of this male–female cooperation that has a broad cross-cultural grounding is not the polite cooperation of professional colleagues but the solidarity of extended kinship groups. Incest taboos that forbid sex among members of the same family may also be generalized to more formal tribal subdivisions such as clans. Mutual interest in the survival and success of the clan can promote both vertical and horizontal cohesion that binds the primary group together among and across age and status cohorts. Women's propensity to bond with family members should also promote cohesion when this norm is dominant.

MILITARY WOMEN'S EXPERIENCES: A PRELIMINARY SAMPLING

Our overview of how male and female sexual strategies may play out in a military context yields a host of predictions about likely associations. One set of predictions links three normative views (women as intruders, sexual resources, or comrades) with the expected prevalence of different forms of male-on-female sexual assault and consensual heterosexual sex. The other links the sexual behaviors of military men and women with horizontal and vertical cohesion in their units. These hypothesized links are collected in Table 1.

Systematic data that would allow us to test these proposed connections are not yet available. A few studies provide fragments of the picture that suggest we are on the right track. For example, Rosen and colleagues (2003) measured group climate using the company as the unit of analysis. They found that unit-level differences were associated with differences in cohesion and attitudes toward spouses, a measure of respect for pair bonds with mates outside the unit. Sadler, Booth, and Doebbeling (2005) found that the severity of emotional trauma and physical impairment differed with the number of assailants and the number of rapes victims reported; in another study

TABLE 1 Expected Associations Among Unit Norms, Sexual Behaviors, and Unit Cohesion

	Expected impact of normative views of women on behavior pursued			Expected impact of behavior on cohesion		
				Horizontal		Vertical
Sexual behavior	Intruders	Sexual resource	Colleague/ comrade	Males	Mixed sex	Males
Male sexual behaviors						
Sexual assault						
Individual attack	▲	▲	▼		▼	
Collective attack	▲		▼	▲	▼	
Rank coercion		▲			▼	▼
Consensual						
Pair bond						
Within unit	▼	▲	▼	▼	▼	
Across ranks		▲	▼		▼	▼
Outside unit only		▲	▲	▲	▲	
Promiscuous						
Within unit	▲	▲	▼	▲	▼	
Outside unit		▲		▲	▼	
Female sexual behaviors						
Consensual						
Pair bond						
Within unit	▲	▲	▼	▼	▼	
Across ranks	▲	▲	▼		▼	▼
Outside unit			▲			
Promiscuous						
Multiple partner						
Within unit	▲	▲	▼	▲	▼	
Outside unit					▼	

Notes. ▲ = expected increase in attractiveness of behavior and in cohesion; ▼ = expected decrease in attractiveness of behavior and in cohesion.

(Sadler et al., 2003), many women reported choosing the sexual strategy of pairing to lessen their risk of MSA.

For this article, we have drawn on the naturalistic data of narratives to develop a preliminary typology of military women's experiences that fleshes out our framework. Our goal is to explore how the components of cultural norms and sexual behaviors by both men and women intersect in the experiences of military women. Our typology distinguishes among individual, dyadic, and collective encounters and discriminates among experiences that are physically forced upon women, those that the women are coerced into, and those that they choose.

Physical Attack: Individual Assault and Gang Rape

A woman may be sexually assaulted by an individual attacker or by multiple attackers. Individual assaults that develop after a woman rejects a man's sexual advances fit the sexual resource conception. Gang rape and more physically violent individual attacks fit with the woman as intruder conception. The sexual resource view may also play a role, as norms of militarized masculinity may promote gang rapes as a bonding experience for primary groups (Wood, 2009) analogous to collective visits to prostitutes. Among women reporting one or more completed rapes during their military service, 14% had been gang-raped (Sadler et al., 2003, p. 266).

Sergeant Kayla Williams, who served in a military intelligence company, provided an example of an individual assault by a fellow soldier during a night shift in Iraq. Until this event occurred, Williams had felt that she had been accepted as a fellow soldier by the men in her unit (woman as comrade norm).

> It's dark, but not so dark that I can't decipher at some point that Rivers' pants are open. That he's got one hand on his penis. And then suddenly, he's also got one hand on my arm. He's pulling me pretty firmly toward him, maneuvering my hand toward his crotch.
>
> "What the fuck—"
>
> I pull back hard, but Rivers is strong. He's still grabbing my arm, preventing me from leaving.
>
> "No," I say. "No, no, no, no, no. Let me go. Let me the fuck go."
>
> "What?" He is genuinely puzzled sounding. "Nobody has to know." (Williams, 2005, p. 207)

Rivers relents and apologizes the next day, acknowledging "I was totally out of line" (p. 208). In debating whether to report the incident, Williams questioned whether the other men would support her or Rivers. In the end, she spoke informally with a superior and Rivers was reassigned, but the event alienated Williams from most of her fellow soldiers.

Williams's account makes clear that Rivers was hoping for consensual sex and was not trying to drive her away. After the attack, Williams did withdraw psychologically from her unit. She also let the other men believe (incorrectly) that she had pair bonded with a trusted male friend within her unit. Tracing the sequence in Table 1, Rivers categorized Williams as a sexual resource, consistent with individual sexual assault, which prompted Rivers to promote the appearance of a pair bond and damaged horizontal cohesion between Williams and the men in her unit.

The woman as intruder view is prominent in gang rape accounts, as exemplified by the experience of staff sergeant and decorated combat medic Sharon Mixon. Mixon reported being drugged and gang-raped by U.S. soldiers during Operation Desert Storm:

> "I woke up face down on a cot. I was being held down. And there were six men taking turns raping me," recalls Mixon. "They told me that if I told anybody that they would kill me. I went and told the [military police] anyway. And they told me the same thing." (Leung, 2005)

Mixon's rapists told her that she should have "expected" such treatment from them. Solidarity among the rapists and the military police suggests strong horizontal cohesion among the men. The threats to kill her indicate that she was viewed primarily as an intruder who threatened the integrity of the male-bonded group (see Table 1). It appears that in their minds, this perceived threat outweighed the value she was contributing as a combat medic.

Rank-Based Coercion

Accounts of rank-based coercion (also called "command rape"; Corbett, 2007) suggest it is an individual form of MSA in line with viewing women as a sexual resource. Soviet veteran Vera Ivanovna Malakhova reported how the power of rank constrained her response to unwanted advances by a commissar: "I remember that I was shaking all over. If things had been different I would have slapped him in the face. But here I couldn't, he was my superior" (Engel, 1999, p. 144).

Army Specialist Suzanne Swift, who went AWOL rather than return for another tour of duty in Iraq, attributed her PTSD to the combined stresses of combat and command rape. Swift was coerced into sexual relations with her squad leader that lasted 4 months (Corbett, 2007). In a study by Sadler and colleagues (2003, p. 267), 40% of women veterans who had been raped said that they did not report the assault because the perpetrator was a ranking officer in their chain of command.

Command rape should heighten tensions in the hierarchy between the rapist and subordinate men who may view the woman as a comrade and see a superior abusing one of their peers. However, other soldiers may also interpret the woman's behavior as that of a "slut" who is seeking advantage via a consensual dyadic relationship. The latter interpretation should damage horizontal cohesion between men and women in the unit. Either interpretation should damage vertical cohesion (see Table 1).

Consensual Sex

Consensual sex can be dyadic or collective and fits the women as sexual resource view. Women who get sexually involved with male soldiers may view the men as a sexual resource, may be trading sex for other benefits such as protection or special treatment, or both. This category includes all voluntary sexual relationships.

The "mobile field wives" attached to Soviet officers at the front during World War II provides an example of dyadic relations that offered benefits to both parties. As Vera Ivanovna Malakhova recalled, "Sexual relations occurred at the front: legitimate, illegitimate, it existed . . . it degraded people and elevated people and saved their lives" (Engel, 1999, p. 146). Women like Malakhova who remained uninvolved resented the field wives as contributing to the image of frontline women as "whores": "We conducted ourselves honorably and disliked the PPZh [the Russian acronym for mobile field wives]. They had privileges" (Engel, 1999, p. 146).

According to many military women, "slut" is a slur used liberally by U.S. military men, often with little connection to actual sexual behavior. "You're a bitch, a slut or a dyke—or you're married, but even if you're married, you're still probably one of the three" (Myers, 2009). However, some women do choose sexual promiscuity as a way to connect with multiple men in or outside their units. Williams (2005, p. 18) reported, "Take this one girl. I heard from reliable sources in Iraq that she gave head to every guy in her unit. . . . I heard it from guys who were there . . . this particular girl got caught in the act . . . More than once." Williams and other military women who wish to be viewed as fellow soldiers and comrades resent sexually promiscuous women who make it tougher "for the rest of us females to get our work done without having guys insinuate that blow jobs was part of our Advanced Individual Training" (p. 19). Although collective sex may heighten horizontal cohesion among the men, it creates friction among military women and can damage horizontal cohesion among men and women in mixed units because of unwelcome assumptions that make it harder for women to be accepted as professional colleagues.

Along with sexual pleasure, military women may use sex to gain acceptance, attention, and, according to Williams (2005), lots of special favors that "could make your load while deployed a whole lot lighter" (p. 20). Military women may seek out protective arrangements with men via sexual relationships. A recent study of veterans found that 27% of women reported getting involved in a relationship with a man as a defensive strategy against sexual harassment and assault (Sadler et al., 2003, p. 266). This protection is liable to be most effective when pairing with either a man within the same unit or an officer in the direct line of command who has power over the other men from whom the women seeks protection. The former choice should damage horizontal cohesion among males, and the latter choice should damage vertical cohesion (see Table 1). Both should damage horizontal cohesion among men and women in mixed units.

Collegial Nonsexual

Collegial nonsexual relationships among men and women are what Rosen and colleagues (2003) called "ungendered professionalism." Instead of being viewed as a sex resource or intruders, women are viewed by the men as comrades-in-arms. A welcome counterpoint to the stories of sexual assault are the narratives of military women who work closely and effectively with men. Marine Corps Lance Corporal Chrissy DeCaprio gained professional acceptance as a fellow Marine by demonstrating her high level of competence.

> She started as a gunner and later was promoted to team leader. The artillery Marines weren't used to working with women because their military occupational specialty is closed to females. . . . One male gunner thought he was the best shot . . . until DeCaprio appeared on the scene and showed him up. (Holmstedt, 2007, p. 143)

While she was serving at the front during World War II, Malakhova also had many positive experiences with men in her unit. Although officers harassed and assaulted her, she felt safe among the rank-and-file male soldiers, even when sleeping among them in the trenches. Soldiers had a "chaste" attitude to the women, she concluded. "To them, we were all 'little sister,' " she said (Engel, 1999, pp. 143–144). As sisters, servicewomen were off limits sexually, as sex would violate an incest taboo. As a male Soviet veteran put it: "We did not look upon them as women . . . You don't marry your own sister, do you?" (Engel, 1999, pp. 143–144).

CONCLUSION

The evolutionary lens focused our attention on the interplay between the imperatives of military effectiveness and the sometimes compatible, sometimes clashing strategies of military men and women. Our evolutionary framework suggests that sexual tensions per se cannot be erased because they are structural, based on thousands of years of natural and sexual selection. Yet male sexual coercion of women in the military varies greatly in different circumstances and contexts, so it is *not* an "immutable fact of nature" (Drea & Wallen, 2003; Geary, 1998; Goldstein, 2001; Gowaty, 2003; Smuts, 1992, p. 24). Many women in the military are sexually assaulted, and many are not. A minority of men will rape if given the opportunity, and the majority will not. Merrill, Thomsen, Gold, and Milner (2001) reported that 10%–11% of Navy recruits had raped someone before enlisting. In a civilian context, rapists are considered criminals at high risk of reoffending, especially if they are confident of getting away with the crime. The same should be true in the military. Along with the impact of unit norms and leadership, the presence of an experienced rapist in a unit should increase the risk of MSA. Hence, the prevalence of assaults should exhibit clusters and concentrations rather than be distributed evenly.

The identification of sexualized workplaces as a risk factor for MSA highlights the generalized impact of a salient normative view of women as a sexual resource (Sadler et al., 2003). Complete abstinence from heterosexual activity is probably the strongest signal that a woman does not want to be viewed by men as a potential sexual partner. However, as Williams (2005) commented, "Sex is not specifically prohibited for deployed soldiers . . . So get real. The Army is not a monastery" (p. 21).

A non-fraternization policy applied at the squad or platoon level may be a realistic way to promote a brother–sister model of professional cooperation within one's primary unit without creating impractical restrictions on consensual sex. Declaring within-unit sex off limits in the interest of unit cohesion is analogous to non-fraternization policies that protect the integrity of command by forbidding relations between officers and enlisted personnel. As Morris (1996, p. 756) noted, the definition of *unit* should take into account both what size of group operates as the primary unit of cohesion and the reality that the smaller the number of colleagues who are included in the incest taboo, the more likely the policy will be observed. Just as non-fraternization policies are not completely successful in preventing relations between officers and enlisted, incest prohibitions will not be invariably honored. However, positive brother–sister norms such as those reported by Malakhova on the front lines in World War II show that this approach can be embraced by ordinary soldiers.

Much of the literature on war and gender focuses on the power of male alliances and the androcentric military organization but fails to recognize female autonomy and choice. Gendered dynamics are just that—*gendered*. Individual behavior and group dynamics involve *both* men and women who base their decisions on the relative attractiveness (or degrees of unattractiveness) of available choices within varying contexts. Norms, policies, and practices can affect how men who are prone to rape assess the possible career risks of assaulting fellow soldiers. They can affect the likelihood that military men will be vigilant against all threats to their fellow soldiers, including the threat of MSA. Based on evolutionary logic, traditional military culture, existing studies (e.g., Morris, 1996; Rosen et al., 2003), and personal narratives (e.g., Engel, 1999; Williams, 2005), we believe that the prevalence of different forms of MSA should covary with different group norms, contexts, and individual strategies.

A growing literature provides some evidence of a varying prevalence of MSA but at a very poor level of resolution—branches of service (Morris, 1996) or different Reserve components (Street, Stafford, Mahan, & Hendricks, 2008). To systematically test for the predicted associations summarized in Table 1 at a finer level of resolution, we need to measure the prevalence of the three normative views as aspects of culture/climate at the company level, as Rosen and colleagues (2003) did. We also need measures of horizontal and vertical cohesion, data on different forms of sexual assault and on sexual behavior by both men and women at the unit level, and information about the enforcement of policies regarding fraternization and professional relationships. Policy implications will flow from regularities in such data. Demonstrated impacts on vertical and horizontal cohesion can serve as a proxy for the relevance of MSA and consensual sex to military effectiveness.

In civilian society, the threat of retaliation from male relatives can be a potent deterrent to rape. In the military, where women are not surrounded by kin, military men could help deter rape by promoting the brother–sister model within their own immediate unit. This can encourage brotherly vigilance against threats to their military "sisters" from outsiders, and evoking the incest taboo can deter advances from other soldiers within the unit. Unfortunately, brotherly vigilance may not deter attacks by men who are in the direct chain of command for all the men and women in the unit. Such command rape can be especially devastating to a soldier's psychological health and ability to function effectively because of the betrayal involved (Birrell & Freyd, 2006) and can also damage trust in leadership by other soldiers in the unit who know about the attacks.

The role of men and women in leadership positions in establishing and enforcing appropriate norms is critical. The entanglement between gender dynamics and military organization makes the actions of officers particularly important in signaling what behaviors are acceptable. One study found that when officers permit others in their unit to make sexually demeaning comments or gestures in the presence of a military woman, rape is 4 times more likely to occur than when they do not (Sadler et al., 2003, p. 269). Far too many officers are using their rank either as a weapon of sexual coercion or to protect soldiers under their command who are attacking their colleagues. Rooting out this problem will require a transformation of military norms and practices beyond what rank-and-file military men and women can accomplish on their own. Cultural interventions that take into account deep-seated and long-standing conceptions of women as intruders or sexual resources are needed to alter an environment in which sexual assault includes not only individual acts of coercion but also group-based responses to perceived threats to traditional military structures.

Although doubts persist about whether it is wise to include women in combat units (e.g., Browne, 2007), the reality of gender-integrated combat support units on the ground in Iraq and Afghanistan makes it clear that military women have become essential to combat activities. "Iraq has advanced the cause of full integration for women in the Army by leaps and bounds," states Army Colonel Peter R. Mansoor (Alvarez, 2009). Thoughtful theory building, focused data collection, and the implementation of sensible policy recommendations informed by theory and data should help reduce the prevalence of sexual assaults that threaten the cohesion and effectiveness of the gender-integrated units on which the U.S. military increasingly depends.

NOTE

1. The application of evolutionary theory to social behavior continues to provoke lively debate. Although misconceptions persist, most scholars who follow these debates closely have moved beyond "straw man" characterizations toward more substantive discussion. Increased attention to gene–environment interactions has made it clear that neither biological nor environmental factors should be treated as deterministic (see Hrdy, 2000; Hubbard, 1990; Thornhill & Palmer, 2000, for contrasting perspectives). Claims that evolutionary theory is untestable have also become less tenable as studies testing hypotheses derived from evolutionary thinking accumulate (e.g., Buller, 2005; Gowaty, 1997; Wilson, Daly, & Scheib, 1997). Buss and Malamuth (1996) provided a useful integration between feminist and evolutionary perspectives.

REFERENCES

Alvarez, L. (2009, August 15). G.I. Jane breaks the combat barrier. *The New York Times*. Retrieved from http://www.nytimes.com/2009/08/16/us/16women.html

Birrell, P. J., & Freyd, J. J. (2006). Betrayal trauma: Relational models of harm and healing. *Journal of Trauma Practice*, *5*(1), 49–63.

Bourke, J. (2007). *Rape: Sex, violence, history*. Berkeley, CA: Counterpoint.

Brightman, R. (1996). The sexual division of foraging labor: Biology, taboo, and gender politics. *Comparative Studies in Society and History*, *38*, 687–729.

Browne, K. (2007). *Co-ed combat: The new evidence that women should not fight the nation's wars*. New York, NY: Penguin.

Buller, D. J. (2005). *Adapting minds: Evolutionary psychology and the persistent quest for human nature*. Cambridge, MA: MIT Press.

Buss, D. M., & Malamuth, N. M. (1996). *Sex, power, conflict: Evolutionary and feminist perspectives*. Oxford, England: Oxford University Press.

Campbell, A. (2002). *A mind of her own: The evolutionary psychology of women*. Oxford, England: Oxford University Press.

Chagnon, N. A. (1988, February 26). Life histories, blood revenge, and warfare in a tribal population. *Science*, *239*, 985–992.

Corbett, S. (2007, March 18). The women's war. *The New York Times*. Retrieved from http://www.nytimes.com/2007/03/18/magazine/18cover.html?ref=magazine

Daly, M., & Wilson, M. (1978). *Sex, evolution and behaviour*. Boston, MA: Willard Grant.

De Pauw, L. G. (1998). *Battle cries and lullabies: Women in war from prehistory to the present*. Norman: University of Oklahoma Press.

Drea, C. M., & Wallen, K. (2003). Female sexuality and the myth of male control. In C. B. Travis (Ed.), *Evolution, gender, and rape* (pp. 29–60). Cambridge, MA: MIT Press.

Engel, B. A. (1999). The womanly face of war: Soviet women remember World War II. In N. A. Dombrowski (Ed.), *Women and war in the twentieth century: Enlisted with or without consent* (pp. 138–161). New York, NY: Garland.

Enloe, C. H. (2000). *Maneuvers: The international politics of militarizing women's lives*. Berkeley: University of California Press.

Fitzgerald, L. F., Drasgow, F., & Magley, V. J. (1999). Sexual harassment in the armed forces: A test of an integrated model. *Military Psychology*, *11*, 329–343.

Friedman, M. J. (2006). Posttraumatic stress disorder among military returnees from Afghanistan and Iraq. *American Journal of Psychiatry*, *163*, 586–593.

Geary, D. C. (1998). *Male, female: The evolution of human sex differences*. Washington, DC: American Psychological Association.

Goldstein, J. S. (2001). *War and gender: How gender shapes the war system and vice versa*. Cambridge, England: Cambridge University Press.

Gottschall, J. (2004). Explaining wartime rape. *Journal of Sex Research*, *41*(2), 129–136.

Gowaty, P. A. (1997). *Feminism and evolutionary biology: Boundaries, intersections, and frontiers*. New York, NY: Chapman & Hall.

Gowaty, P. A. (2003). Power asymmetries between the sexes, mate preferences, and components of fitness. In C. B. Travis (Ed.), *Evolution, gender, and rape* (pp. 61–86). Cambridge, MA: MIT Press.

Greenbaum, C. W. (1979). The small group under the gun: Uses of small groups in battle conditions. *Journal of Applied Behavioral Science*, *15*, 392–405.

Griffith, J. (1988). Measurement of group cohesion in US army units. *Basic and Applied Social Psychology*, *9*(2), 149–171.

Harned, M. S., Ormerod, A. J., Palmieri, P. A., Collinsworth, L. L., & Reed, M. (2002). Sexual assault and other types of sexual harassment by workplace personnel: A comparison of antecedents and consequences. *Journal of Occupational Health Psychology*, *7*(2), 174–188.

Henry, N., Ward, T., & Hirshberg, M. (2004). A multifactorial model of wartime rape. *Aggression and Violent Behavior*, *9*, 535–562.

Holmstedt, K. A. (2007). *Band of sisters: American women at war in Iraq*. Mechanicsburg, PA: Stackpole Books.

Hrdy, S. B. (2000). *Mother nature: Maternal instincts and how they shape the human species*. New York, NY: Ballantine Books.

Hrdy, S. B. (2009). *Mothers and others: The evolutionary origins of mutual understanding*. Cambridge, MA: Belknap Press.

Hubbard, R. (1990). *The politics of women's biology*. New Brunswick, NJ: Rutgers University Press.

Iasiello, L. V., Wasell, M., Arias, I., Carpenter, A. M., Dunbar, S. K. G., Grant, J. M., . . . Swiatek, S. M. (2009, December). *Report of the Defense Task Force on Sexual Assault in the Military Services* Retrieved from http://www.dtic.mil/dtfsams/docs/11_09docs/DTFSAMS-Rept_Dec09.pdf

Kang, H., Dalager, N., Mahan, C., & Ishii, E. (2005). The role of sexual assault on the risk of PTSD among Gulf War veterans. *Annals of Epidemiology*, *15*, 191–195.

Keeley, L. H. (1997). *War before civilization: The myth of the peaceful savage*. New York, NY: Oxford University Press.

Kimerling, R., Gima, K., Smith, M. W., Street, A., & Frayne, S. (2007). The Veterans Health Administration and military sexual trauma. *American Journal of Public Health*, *97*, 2160–2166.

LeBlanc, S. A. (1999). *Prehistoric warfare in the American southwest*. Salt Lake City: University of Utah Press.

Leung, R. (2005, February 20). Army rape accuser speaks out. *CBS/60 Minutes*. Retrieved from http://www.cbsnews.com/stories/2005/02/17/60minutes/main674791.shtml

Littlewood, R. (1997). Military rape. *Anthropology Today*, *13*(2), 7–16.

Low, B. S. (2001). *Why sex matters: A Darwinian look at human behavior*. Princeton, NJ: Princeton University Press.

Marshall, S. L. A. (1947). *Men against fire: The problem of battle command in future war*. Oxford, England: Infantry Journal Press.

Merrill, L. L., Thomsen, C. J., Gold, S. R., & Milner, J. S. (2001). Childhood abuse and premilitary sexual assault in male navy recruits. *Journal of Consulting and Clinical Psychology*, *69*, 252–261.

Moon, K. H. S. (1997). *Sex among allies: Military prostitution in US-Korea relations*. New York, NY: Columbia University Press.

Morris, M. (1996). By force of arms: Rape, war, and military culture. *Duke Law Journal*, *44*, 651–781.

Murdoch, M., Polusny, M. A., Hodges, J., & O'Brien, N. (2004). Prevalence of in-service and post-service sexual assault among combat and noncombat veterans applying for Department of Veterans Affairs posttraumatic stress disorder disability benefits. *Military Medicine*, *169*, 392–395.

Myers, S. L. (2009, August 16). Living and fighting alongside men, and fitting in. *The New York Times*. Retrieved from http://www.nytimes.com/2009/08/17/us/17women.html

Rosen, L. N., Durand, D. B., Bliese, P. D., Halverson, R. R., Rothberg, J. M., & Harrison, N. L. (1996). Cohesion and readiness in gender-integrated combat service support units: The impact of acceptance of women and gender ratio. *Armed Forces & Society*, *22*, 537–553.

Rosen, L. N., Knudson, K. H., & Fancher, P. (2003). Cohesion and the culture of hypermasculinity in US army units. *Armed Forces & Society*, *29*, 325–351.

Sadler, A. G., Booth, B. M., Cook, B. L., & Doebbeling, B. N. (2003). Factors associated with women's risk of rape in the military environment. *American Journal of Industrial Medicine*, *43*(3), 262–273.

Sadler, A. G., Booth, B. M., & Doebbeling, B. N. (2005). Gang and multiple rapes during military service: Health consequences and health care. *Journal of the American Medical Women's Association*, *60*(1), 33–41.

Seeley, E. A., Gardner, W. L., Pennington, G., & Gabriel, S. (2003). Circle of friends or members of a group? Sex differences in relational and collective attachment to groups. *Group Processes & Intergroup Relations*, *6*(3), 251–263.

Shils, E. A., & Janowitz, M. (1948). Cohesion and disintegration in the Wehrmacht in World War II. *Public Opinion Quarterly*, *12*, 280–315.

Smuts, B. (1992). Male aggression against women: An evolutionary perspective. *Human Nature*, *3*(1), 1–44.

Sosis, R., Kress, H. C., & Boster, J. S. (2007). Scars for war: Evaluating alternative signaling explanations for cross-cultural variance in ritual costs. *Evolution and Human Behavior*, *28*(4), 234–247.

Stiglmayer, A. (1994). *Mass rape: The war against women in Bosnia-Herzegovina*. Lincoln: University of Nebraska Press.

Street, A. E., Stafford, J., Mahan, C. M., & Hendricks, A. (2008). Sexual harassment and assault experienced by reservists during military service: Prevalence and health correlates. *Journal of Rehabilitation Research and Development*, *45*, 409–420.

Suris, A., & Lind, L. (2008). Military sexual trauma: A review of prevalence and associated health consequences in veterans. *Trauma, Violence, & Abuse*, *9*(4), 250–269.

Thornhill, R., & Palmer, C. T. (2000). *A natural history of rape: Biological bases of sexual coercion*. Cambridge, MA: MIT Press.

Trivers, R. L. (1972). Parental investment and sexual selection. In B. Campbell (Ed.), *Sexual selection and the descent of man 1871-1971* (pp. 136–179). Chicago, IL: Aldine.

Trivers, R. L. (1974). Parent-offspring conflict. *American Zoologist*, *14*(1), 249–264.

Van Vugt, M., De Cremer, D., & Janssen, D. P. (2007). Gender differences in cooperation and competition: The male-warrior hypothesis. *Psychological Science*, *18*, 19–23.

Wildschut, T., Pinter, B., Vevea, J. L., Insko, C. A., & Schopler, J. (2003). Beyond the group mind: A quantitative review of the interindividual-intergroup discontinuity effect. *Psychological Bulletin*, *129*, 698–722.

Williams, K. (2005). *Love my rifle more than you: Young and female in the US army*. New York, NY: Norton.

Wilson, M., Daly, M., & Scheib, J. E. (1997). Femicide: An evolutionary psychological perspective. In P. A. Gowaty (Ed.), *Feminism and evolutionary biology: Boundaries, intersections, and frontiers* (pp. 431–465). New York, NY: Chapman & Hall.

Wood, E. J. (2009). Armed groups and sexual violence: When is wartime rape rare? *Politics & Society*, *37*(1), 131–161.

Yaeger, D., Himmelfarb, N., Cammack, A., & Mintz, J. (2006). *DSM-IV* diagnosed posttraumatic stress disorder in women veterans with and without military sexual trauma. *Journal of General Internal Medicine*, *21*, 65–69.

Zihlman, A. L. (1981). Women as shapers of the human adaptation. In F. Dahlberg (Ed.), *Woman the gatherer* (pp. 75–120). New Haven, CT: Yale University Press.

Military Sexual Trauma Research: A Proposed Agenda

CAROLYN B. ALLARD, PhD and SARAH NUNNINK, PhD
Psychology Service, Department of Veterans Affairs Medical Center and Department of Psychiatry, University of California, San Diego, California, USA

AMBER M. GREGORY, BA
Research Service, Department of Veterans Affairs Medical Center, San Diego, California, USA

BRIDGET KLEST, PhD
Department of Veterans Affairs Medical Center, Seattle, Washington, USA

MELISSA PLATT, MA, MS
Department of Psychology, University of Oregon, Eugene, Oregon, USA

Military sexual trauma (MST) is a widespread problem associated with negative psychological and physical health problems. This article presents the current state of MST research and highlights specific areas in need of more focused study. Areas that have produced the greatest body of knowledge include MST prevalence and psychological and physical health correlates. We propose a research agenda based on gaps noted in our research review and empirical and theoretical evidence of issues relevant to but not studied directly in MST populations. We present evidence that MST is qualitatively distinct from other forms of sexual maltreatment in terms of its relational and vocational context as well as the severity

---

Research was conducted at the VA San Diego Healthcare System and University of California, San Diego.

This material is the result of work supported with resources and the use of facilities at the VA San Diego Healthcare Center. No part of this article has been presented or published elsewhere. The views expressed in this article are those of the authors and do not necessarily reflect the position or policy of the Department of Veterans Affairs or the United States government. The authors declare no conflicts of interest or financial relationships related to this research.

of associated psychological distress, examine underexplored gender and sexual issues in MST, and discuss the lack of treatment and prevention studies specific to MST. Specific recommendations are made throughout in an attempt to guide and advance the field.

The prevalence and correlates of sexual abuse, assault, and harassment have been studied extensively since the emergence of literature on this topic in the 1960s. Although earlier accounts of sexual abuse in the military can be found in scientific journals (e.g., Waldfogel & Mueser, 1988), scientific attention was spurred by a 1992 Congressional mandate for the Department of Veterans Affairs to treat distress related to military sexual trauma (MST). The term *military sexual trauma* was coined to capture the different forms of sexual maltreatment reported by military personnel and is defined as follows: "sexual harassment that is threatening in character, or physical assault of a sexual nature that occurred while the victim was in the military, regardless of geographic location of the trauma, gender of victim, or the relationship to the perpetrator" (Veterans' Benefits U.S. Code, Section 1720D, 1992). *MST* is used accordingly in this article, whereas *sexual assault* is used to refer specifically to unwanted physical contact involving sexual body parts, and *sexual harassment* denotes unsolicited verbal or physical contact of a sexual nature (e.g., pressure for sexual favors, unwanted touching of nonsexual body parts).

Following the mandate, 61% of Veterans Affairs medical centers had sexual trauma treatment teams by 1995 (Suris, Davis, Kashner, Gillaspy, & Petty, 1998), and MST continues to receive research attention. Yet much remains unknown. The aims of this article are to highlight gaps in research and to propose a research agenda to continue to improve MST conceptualization and intervention efforts.

To examine the available body of MST research and identify the gaps in knowledge, we conducted a systematic search and categorization of studies pertaining to MST. Using PsycINFO and MEDLINE searches for peer-reviewed journal articles published up to December 2009 (with keyword combinations including *military* or *veteran* and *sexual assault*, *sexual harassment*, or *sexual trauma*) and reviewing reference lists within the articles uncovered by this search, we identified 74 MST articles (marked with asterisks in the reference list). The main characteristics of the MST articles are presented in Table 1. Research has largely focused on identifying the prevalence and incidence of abuse and psychological and physical health correlates, which we review first, noting any remaining gaps in knowledge in these areas. We follow with a series of questions that are in need of much more research attention if experts are to have a thorough understanding of the impact of MST and how to prevent it and its aftermath.

TABLE 1 Military Sexual Trauma Articles by Type of Study and Gender Composition of Results

				Both genders	
Category	*N*	Female only	Male only	Gender-specific data reported	No gender-specific data reported
Prevalence	52	32	1	16	3
		Bostock & Daley (2007); Butterfield et al. (1998); Campbell et al. (2006); Campbell & Raja (2005); Carney et al. (2003); Castillo et al. (2002); Chang et al. (2001); Coyle et al. (1996); David et al. (2006); DeRoma et al. (2003); Dutra et al. (2001); Fontana & Rosenheck (1998); Fontana et al. (1997); Frayne et al. (1999, 2003); Hankin et al. (1999); Harned et al. (2002); Himmelfarb et al. (2006); Katz et al. (2007); McCall-Hosenfeld et al. (2009); Murdoch & Nichol (1995); Newell et al. (1995); Sadler et al. (2000, 2001, 2003, 2004); Schnurr et al. (2007); Skinner et al. (2000); Suris et al. (2004, 2007); Wolfe et al. (1998); Yaeger et al. (2006)	Smith et al. (1999)	Fitzgerald et al. (1999); Kang et al. (2004); Kimerling et al. (2007); Magley et al. (1999); Martin et al. (1998, 2000); Murdoch et al. (2003, 2004, 2006, 2007); Rosen & Martin (1998a); Shipherd et al. (2009); Stark et al. (2002); Street et al. (2007, 2008); Vogt et al. (2005)	Magley & Shupe (2005); Monson et al. (2006); Rauch et al. (2009)

Mental health correlates	37	20	1	12	4
		Butterfield et al. (1998); Campbell & Raja (2005); Castillo et al. (2002); Chang et al. (2001); DeRoma et al. (2003); Dutra et al. (2001); Fontana & Rosenheck (1998); Fontana et al. (1997); Hankin et al. (1999); Himmelfarb et al. (2006); Katz et al. (2007); McCall-Hosenfeld et al. (2009); Murdoch & Nichol (1995); Sadler et al. (2000, 2004); Skinner et al. (2000); Suris et al. (2004, 2007); Wolfe et al. (1998); Yaeger et al. (2006)	Smith et al. (1999)	Harned & Fitzgerald (2002); Kang et al. (2004); Kimerling et al. (2007); Magley et al. (1999); Martin et al. (2000); Murdoch et al. (2006, 2007); O'Brien et al. (2008); Shipherd et al. (2009); Street et al. (2007, 2008); Vogt et al. (2005)	Bergman et al. (2002); Monson et al. (2006); Murdoch et al. (2003); Rauch et al. (2009)
Physical health correlates	15	9	0	6	0
		Campbell et al. (2006); Frayne et al. (1999); Frayne et al. (2003); McCall-Hosenfeld et al. (2009); Murdoch & Nichol (1995); Sadler et al. (2000, 2004); Skinner et al. (2000); Suris et al. (2007)		Harned & Fitzgerald (2002); Kimerling et al. (2007); Martin et al. (2000); Murdoch et al. (2007); Shipherd et al. (2009); Street et al. (2008)	

(*Continued*)

TABLE 1 (Continued)

Category	*N*	Female only	Male only	Both genders: Gender-specific data reported	Both genders: No gender-specific data reported
Health care utilization	7	6	0	0	1
		Campbell & Raja (2005); Coyle et al. (1996); Murdoch & Nichol (1995); Sadler et al. (2004); Skinner et al. (2000); Suris et al. (2004)			Suris et al. (1998)
Treatment outcome	7	3	1	1	2
		David et al. (2006); Katz et al. (2008); Schnurr et al. (2007)	Waldfogel & Mueser (1988)	O'Brien et al. (2008)	Monson et al. (2006); Rauch et al. (2009)
Literature review	3	2	0	1	0
		Goldzweig et al. (2006); Zinzow et al. (2007)		Suris & Lind (2008)	
Other	12	Culbertson & Rosenfeld (2002); David et al. (2004); M. E. Hall et al. (2007); Houser (2007); Kelley et al. (2005); Leskela et al. (2001); Raiha (1983); Ritchie (1998); Rosen & Martin (1998b); Valente & Wright (2007); Vogt et al. (2007); Young (1995)			

MST PREVALENCE

Exact prevalence rates of MST have been difficult to gauge, given variation across study methodologies, including in source and characteristics of the sample, data collection strategy, and definition and assessment of MST. Consistent with prior reviews (Goldzweig, Balekian, Rolón, Yano, & Shekelle, 2006; Suris & Lind, 2008; Zinzow, Grubaugh, Monnier, Suffoletta-Maierle, & Frueh, 2007), we found that most prevalence studies are of actual or threatened sexual assault and report rates ranging from 22% to 45%. Lower prevalence rates have been reported for men and in studies only asking about rape, whereas higher rates have been found in treatment-seeking samples and when full MST definitions and/or sexual harassment experiences are included.

The prevalence of MST is notably similar to lifetime prevalence rates of sexual assault and harassment in the general population (e.g., Norris, 1992; Tjaden & Thoennes, 2000; U.S. Merit Systems Protection Board, 1995). Given that MST occurs within a restricted time period (typically 2 to 6 years of service), the incidence of sexual maltreatment appears to be higher for individuals in the military than in civilian life. Directly comparing female veteran and civilian reports of sexual victimization, Schultz, Bell, Naugle, and Polusny (2006) found significantly higher rates of rape in veterans (49%) than civilians (22%). Furthermore, sexual assaults are underreported in the general population (Friedman, Samet, Roberts, Hudlin, & Hans, 1992; Jenkins & Dambrot, 1987; Mynatt & Allgeier, 1990; Widom & Morris, 1997; Williams, 1994), and contextual factors of a military environment suggest a more profound problem of underreporting in military populations, as we discuss in a later section of this article.

MST CORRELATES

Many studies have found MST to be a strong predictor of psychological distress that manifests in various and complex ways. The most frequently measured forms of distress associated with MST are posttraumatic stress disorder (PTSD), other anxiety and depression symptoms, and poor functioning (for more detailed reviews, see Goldzweig et al., 2006; Suris & Lind, 2008; Zinzow et al., 2007). Growing evidence about the varied and complex presentations of MST-related distress and functioning difficulties suggests that more careful investigation in this area is needed.

For example, complications in sexual functioning following sexual assault are a common complaint yet are understudied as sequelae and intervention targets in MST survivors. In the civilian sexual assault literature, survivors frequently report problems with sexual dysfunction and decreased sexual satisfaction (e.g., Bartoi & Kinder, 1998; Mackey et al.,

1991), including fear, disdain or avoidance of sexual intimacy, and arousal and desire problems. Among female veterans, MST has been linked to decreased sexual satisfaction (McCall-Hosenfeld, Liebschutz, Spiro, & Seaver, 2009; Skinner et al., 2000). In one of the few studies of sexual functioning in male survivors of sexual trauma, 8% of male MST victims reported being fearful of sex, 7% reported decreased sexual interest, and 8% reported fewer pleasurable sexual relations (Siegel, Golding, Stein, Burnam, & Sorenson, 1990). O'Brien, Gaher, Pope, and Smiley (2008) found that male veterans with MST histories exhibited more persistent sexual problems than women. It is important to note that post-assault sexual problems appear to be resistant to spontaneous remission and particularly enduring (Becker, Skinner, Abel, & Cichon, 1986; Burgess & Holmstrom, 1979; Ellis, Calhoun, & Atkeson, 1980). More research is needed on the impact of MST on sexual functioning and other potentially under-detected and under-addressed difficulties faced by both men and women to improve understanding of the impact of MST and to inform intervention efforts.

Another consistent finding is the association between MST history and medical or physical health complaints. Individuals reporting MST experience a greater number of current physical symptoms, more impaired health status, and more chronic health problems than those reporting no MST experiences (see reviews by Goldzweig et al., 2006; Suris & Lind, 2008; Zinzow et al., 2007). Specifically, pelvic pain, menstrual problems, back pain, headaches, gastrointestinal symptoms, chronic fatigue, and cardiovascular risk factors (obesity, smoking, sedentary lifestyle) are more likely in individuals reporting MST than those not reporting MST (e.g., Frayne, Skinner, Sullivan, & Freund, 2003; Stein et al., 2004). Increased utilization of medical services has been found among sexual assault survivors compared to those without such histories (e.g., Kilpatrick, 1992; Stein et al., 2004). Compared to civilian sexual trauma, MST has also been associated with poor physical health and low satisfaction with one's health (Suris, Lind, Kashner, & Borman, 2007). However, controlling for childhood sexual abuse resulted in no association between MST and health care utilization (Suris, Lind, Kashner, Borman, & Petty, 2004). Continued investigation of potential modulators of MST correlates, such as prior trauma, may uncover potential prevention and treatment targets.

Although it is often assumed that the traumatic element of MST lies in actual assaults, sexual harassment does appear to be associated with deleterious mental health consequences in and of itself (Harned & Fitzgerald, 2002; Harned, Ormerod, Palmieri, Collinsworth, & Reed, 2002; Murdoch, Polusny, Hodges, & Cowper, 2006; Street, Stafford, Mahan, & Hendricks, 2008). More careful assessment of MST allowing for the distinction between assault and harassment is needed in order to contribute further to this line of research.

IS MST COMPARABLE TO OTHER SEXUAL TRAUMA?

Although the more abundant research on civilian sexual assault and harassment may be applicable to MST in many ways, it cannot be exclusively relied upon. It can be deduced from non-military-specific research that MST is likely to result in serious negative consequences. Sexual assault is one of the strongest predictors of posttraumatic distress among traumatic experiences (Kessler, Sonnega, Bromet, Hughes, & Nelson, 1995), including military-related traumas like combat (Fontana & Rosenheck, 1998; Katz, Bloor, Cojucar, & Draper, 2007; Wolfe et al., 1998). However, there is also evidence that MST is even more deleterious than civilian sexual trauma in that it has been associated with increased risk for PTSD relative to civilian sexual trauma (Himmelfarb, Yaeger, & Mintz, 2006; Suris et al., 2004, 2007). Researchers have proposed individual, trauma-related, and contextual factors as contributors to MST's relatively more insidious nature compared to other sexual trauma.

One individual factor found to predict greater posttraumatic distress is having experienced multiple traumatic events (King, King, & Foy, 1996; King, King, Foy, Keane, & Fairbank, 1999; Suliman et al., 2009; Testa, VanZile-Tamsen, & Livingston, 2007). This risk appears to be especially prevalent in military personnel who report high rates of trauma before, during, and after their military involvement (e.g., Fontana & Rosenheck, 1998; King et al., 1999; Murdoch, Polusny, Hodges, & O'Brien, 2004). Also noteworthy is that military personnel are more likely than civilians to report lifetime histories of sexual trauma (Merrill et al., 1998; Sadler, Booth, Mengeling, & Doebbeling, 2004; Schultz et al., 2006).

Trauma-related factors may also explain the relatively heightened risk of posttraumatic distress related to MST. Interpersonal trauma is associated with more severe psychological presentation compared to non-interpersonal trauma (Bremner, Southwick, Johnson, Yehuda, & Charney, 1993; Duncan, 2004; Gahm, Lucenko, Retzlaff, & Fukada, 2007; Roth, Newman, Pelcovitz, van der Kolk, & Mandel, 1997; van der Kolk, Roth, Pelcovitz, Sunday, & Spinazzola, 2005). In addition, the closeness of the relationship between victim and perpetrator has been associated with increased dissociation (Chu & Dill, 1990; Plattner et al., 2003), depression (Freyd, Klest, & Allard, 2005), and PTSD symptoms (Allard, 2009), as well as impaired reasoning regarding interpersonal relationships (DePrince, 2005), disrupted memory for the abuse (Freyd, DePrince, & Zurbriggen, 2001), and nondisclosure of abuse (Foynes, Freyd, & DePrince, 2009). Freyd (1996) proposed that the impact of interpersonal trauma is greatest when the victim is dependent upon the perpetrator because this creates conflict between adaptive responses to betrayal and the need to maintain attachment to the relied-upon other. This scenario applies to MST experiences, as most MST is perpetrated by fellow service members (Department of Defense, 2009; Sadler, Booth, Cook, & Doebbeling,

2003), many of whom depend upon one another for their very survival. Further study of the role of betrayal in MST outcomes is thus warranted.

Contextual factors posited to contribute to the more deleterious impact of MST compared to nonmilitary sexual victimization include continued exposure to the perpetrator long after the sexual abuse, the power differential inherent in the military rank system, issues related to unit cohesion, and limitations in social resources and support (Kimerling, Gima, Smith, Street, & Frayne, 2007; Steury, Spencer, & Parkinson, 2004; Suris & Lind, 2008; Tarrier & Humphreys, 2003). Continued exposure to the perpetrator and the inescapable nature of enlistment may contribute to a chronic threat of abuse. The power hierarchy of the military and the pressures of unit cohesion may present obstacles to reporting abuses and pursuing and obtaining justice, as already mentioned. Awareness and discussion of MST perpetrated by a coworker or superior officer in the same or related unit may be avoided for fear of disrupting the focus on military duties, leadership, and cohesion, which could leave the unit members more vulnerable to being killed in combat. Moreover, the context of being stationed away from home or deployed results in limited access to primary support systems; many military responses to MST disclosures have been described as unsupportive at best and victim-blaming and punishing at worst (Fontana & Rosenheck, 1998). Veterans have noted more frequent discouragement from filing official reports, more frequent minimizing of the seriousness of the assault, and more frequent refusals to take reports or pursue the matter when sexual trauma was reported to military officials compared to civilian officials, and these types of responses were associated with posttraumatic distress symptoms (Campbell & Raja, 1999). Future research needs to test these proposed individual, trauma-related, and contextual mediators and moderators of MST's impact on well-being.

ARE THERE GENDER DIFFERENCES IN MST?

The risk of MST exposure differs by gender, with consistently higher rates reported in women than in men. Less than half of the MST articles we found reported gender-specific prevalence rates (see Table 1). Reported rates of MST in men range from <1% to 31%. Although research is limited, men and women appear to be differently impacted by MST. Kimerling et al. (2007) found that MST in both genders was related to dissociative and personality disorders, but it was most strongly related to PTSD and eating disorders in women and to bipolar and psychotic symptoms in men. MST has been associated with obesity, weight loss, and hypothyroidism in women, and with AIDS in men (Frayne et al., 2003). There is some evidence that men may be more negatively impacted by MST than women. Civilian male rape victims may be at higher risk than women for problems concerning gender identity, sexual orientation ambiguity, and anger dysregulation (see review by Leskela, Dieperink, & Kok, 2001). Men with MST histories have exhibited greater levels and persistence of PTSD and other psychiatric symptoms, poorer perceived health, and poorer functioning compared to women (Murdoch, Pryor, Polusny, & Gackstetter, 2007; O'Brien et al., 2008; Shipherd, Pineles, Gradus, & Resick, 2009; Street, Gradus, Stafford, & Kelly, 2007).

Murdoch and colleagues (2007) noted that because men outnumber women in the armed forces, there may actually be more MST impacted men than women. The high value given to traditional male roles in the military is likely influential in the male experience of MST. As highlighted by Murdoch and her colleagues (2004, 2007), hyper-masculinity is common within the military and is incongruent with the stereotyped identity of a sexual assault victim (weak, feminine). The need for research that directly assesses masculine identity, powerlessness, shame, and sexual identity using psychometrically sound measures in male MST populations is ostensible.

ARE EMPIRICALLY SUPPORTED TREATMENTS EFFECTIVE IN MST POPULATIONS?

A review of studies of treatment for sexual assault related distress in women found the most empirical support for Prolonged Exposure (PE; Foa, Hembree, & Rothbaum, 2007) and Cognitive Processing Therapy (CPT; Resick & Schnicke, 1992), and some support for the efficacy of Stress Inoculation Training and Eye Movement Desensitization and Reprocessing (Vickerman & Margolin, 2009). Currently, the VA is "rolling out" (training staff in and including in their best practices guidelines) the evidence based PTSD treatments. As a result, these treatments are increasingly being offered to veterans experiencing MST related distress, although actual utilization rates are currently unknown. While many of the treatment outcome studies supporting the efficacy of PE and CPT have included sexual trauma survivors, only two have reported outcomes specific to MST survivors. The unique combination of stressors faced by MST survivors and the potential gender differences noted previously mean that treatment outcomes in other trauma populations are not necessarily applicable to MST populations. Of additional concern is that an analysis of clinical trial effect sizes revealed a less robust treatment outcome for military populations compared to nonmilitary samples (Cason, Grubaugh, & Resick, 2002).

Monson and colleagues (2006) conducted a randomized clinical trial with 60 veterans, including 10 individuals with MST related PTSD, and found significant reductions in PTSD symptoms for those receiving cognitive processing therapy compared to those on the waitlist using intention-to-treat analyses, but results were not presented separately for the MST subsample. PE was found to be effective in reducing PTSD symptoms and diagnosis in a sample of 284 active duty and veteran women, the majority of whom (73%) endorsed MST (among the mean of 10 different trauma types reported by this sample; Schnurr et al., 2007). Findings specific to MST related distress were not reported but MST was tested and not supported as a modifier of the treatment effect. Over fifty percent of the intent-to-treat sample in this study continued to meet diagnostic criteria for PTSD at posttreatment, and at 3 and 6 month followup (60% for the intent-to-treat sample). In contrast, over one-third of participants receiving PE and CPT retained PTSD diagnosis per Vickerman and Margolin's (2009) review of treatments for sexual assault in women. Also noteworthy, the effect size obtained (d = 0.80) was smaller than for other PE clinical trials in non-veterans. Another Clinical trial of PE included and reported outcomes specific to the two veterans with MST histories (out of a sample of 10), both of whom experienced pre/post reductions in PTSD and depression symptoms but also continued to have scores above the cutoff for PTSD on the assessment measures (Rauch et al., 2009).

Four studies reporting outcomes of other types of treatments that included participants with MST related distress also show promising results with limited inferential value because of small sample sizes, lack of a control comparison, and/or incomplete treatment description. Both men and women ($N = 175$) showed pre/post improvements in MST related PTSD symptoms following a 7-week residential treatment including intensive exposure-based group therapy, psychoeducation, coping skills training, and recreational and wellness activities (O'Brien et al., 2008). No loss of diagnosis or remission rates were reported in this study. A feasibility study of a "reprocessing" treatment involving some cognitive restructuring and imaginal exposure reported significant pre/post reductions in negative cognitions following the intervention but did not measure PTSD symptoms and did not present outcomes specific to the 7 (out of 17) participants with MST histories (Katz, Snetter, Robinson, Hewitt, & Cojucar, 2008). David, Simpson, and Cotton (2006) found significant reductions in PTSD and depression symptoms in 10 women with MST histories up to 6 months after a self-defense training that incorporated exposure and cognitive restructuring. Finally, Waldfogel and Mueser (1988) gave a case presentation of a male veteran with MST related PTSD, auditory hallucinations, and paranoid delusions who was asymptomatic 16 months after completing psychotherapy involving imaginal exposure. These limited findings suggest that veterans who experience MST related posttraumatic distress stand to benefit from some forms of therapy, but clearly more systematic treatment outcome research in MST samples is needed.

TREATMENT ATTRITION

No investigation of treatment completion has been conducted with MST survivors. Attrition rates in PTSD treatment studies have ranged from 0% to 54% (Schottenbauer, Glass, Arnkoff, Tendick, & Gray, 2008), with an average of 35.2% (Sharf, 2008). Dropout rates in non-research clinical practice can be higher than those reported in clinical trials (Persons, Burns, & Perloff, 1988; Steel et al., 2000; Waller, 1997), in part because of fewer resources for follow-up contact. Considering the highest attrition rate in PTSD studies, Zayfert and colleagues (2005) deduced an expected clinical dropout rate of 80%. It is therefore essential to identify predictors of dropout in an effort to develop interventions that address them more successfully.

Lower income and unemployment predict PTSD treatment attrition in some studies (e.g., Matthieu & Ivanoff, 2006). Compared to treatment completers, individuals who drop out of trauma-related treatment tend to be more symptomatic and/or functionally impaired at pretreatment (e.g., Bryant et al., 2007; Zayfert et al., 2005), to have higher alcohol consumption (Difede et al., 2007), and to have received more previous psychological treatment (Marks, Lovell, Noshirvani, Livanou, & Thrasher, 1998; Matthieu & Ivanoff, 2006). The need for additional research on treatment completion and outcomes in MST populations is evident.

WHAT ABOUT THE PREVENTION OF MST?

MST prevention research is also sparse, which is concerning given that military personnel are not only more likely to experience sexual trauma but also more likely to perpetrate sexual assaults compared to their civilian counterparts. Whereas a nationally representative survey of college students found that 4% of men reported ever having perpetrated rape (G. C. N. Hall, Hirschman, Graham, & Zaragoza, 1993), 10%–12% of male U.S. Navy recruits reported having raped a woman before entering military service (Merrill, Thomsen, Gold, & Milner, 2001).

Increasing understanding of sex offender behavior and military social climate factors that potentially contribute to MST may facilitate the development of effective prevention efforts. To this end, Vogt, Bruce, Street, and Stafford (2007) surveyed more than 2,000 reservists and national guards and found that poorer attitudes toward women predicted tolerance of sexual harassment and were more likely in men, ethnic majority members, and Marines. An earlier study revealed an association between negative attitudes toward women, including a lack of acceptance of women as equals in the Army, and tolerance of sexual harassment (Rosen & Martin, 1998b). Other investigations of predictors of MST have been focused more on an individual level. A possible risk factor for sexual trauma is substance abuse (Shannon, Logan, Cole, & Walker, 2008). Rosen and Martin (1998a) found that childhood sexual and physical abuse predicted sexual revictimization and perpetration and that both victimization and perpetration were predictors of poor psychological well-being for both male and female Army soldiers. These predictors of MST point to promising prevention foci.

The Navy's Sexual Assault Victim Intervention program was developed to address some of the empirically identified and theorized predictors of MST and includes training programs to increase sexual assault awareness. No data are yet available on the effectiveness of this program in terms of prevention, but the program was rated by sailors as satisfactory and as contributing to increased job concentration and enhanced health and safety (Kelley, Schwerin, Farrar, & Lane, 2005). After surveying female veterans who believed that personal safety/self-defense training would increase their competence against future assaults, David, Cotton, Simpson, and Weitlauf (2004) developed and tested a self-defense program incorporating cognitive behavioral therapy interventions. Participants reported increases in self-defense self-efficacy from pre- to post-training; however, no data were collected on prevention effectiveness (David et al., 2006).

To summarize, a daunting proportion of service members experience MST at a substantial cost to public health. Our review of the research suggests that there is a need for greater breadth and precision in MST research. One first step toward this aim would be to standardize the definition of MST across research studies. Other recommendations are (a) to measure health and functioning more broadly to capture the full extent of posttraumatic distress experienced by individuals who experience MST and (b) to explore the role of potential modulators of the MST correlates, including other trauma history, gender, victim–perpetrator relationship, and characteristics of the military environment. In addition, systematic treatment effectiveness and efficacy research in MST populations is required. Researchers need to investigate whether the factors that distinguish MST from other sexual abuse play a role in treatment outcomes and whether existing empirically supported treatments adequately address the range of concerns of veterans with distress secondary to MST. Finally, what is most sorely needed is basic and intervention research aimed at primary prevention. Although efforts to raise awareness and provide resources to MST victims have increased in the military over the past 5 years, prevalence rates of MST continue to be alarmingly high. In conclusion, MST researchers are to be commended for bringing to light this prevalent public health concern. Their published findings have propelled national treatment and prevention efforts. Continued and increasingly systematic empirical investigations of the prevalence, risks, and impact of MST and of treatment and prevention efforts are encouraged to improve experts' efforts at addressing MST.

REFERENCES

Allard, C. B. (2009). Prevalence and sequelae of betrayal trauma in a Japanese student sample. *Psychological Trauma: Theory, Research, Practice, and Policy, 1*, 65–77.

Bartoi, M. G., & Kinder, B. N. (1998) The effects of child and adult sexual abuse on adult sexuality. *Journal of Sex and Marital Therapy, 24*, 75–90.

Becker, J. V., Skinner, L. J., Abel, G. G., & Cichon, J. (1986). Level of post assault sexual functioning in rape victims and incest victims. *Archives of Sexual Behavior, 15*, 37–49.

*Bergman, M. E., Langhout, R. D., Palmieri, P. A., Cortina, L. M., & Fitzgerald, L. F. (2002). The (un)reasonableness of reporting: Antecedents and consequences of reporting sexual harassment *Journal of Applied Psychology, 87*, 230–242.

*Bostock, D. J., & Daley, J. G. (2007). Lifetime and current sexual assault and harassment victimization rates of active-duty United States air force women. *Violence Against Women, 13*, 927–944.

Bremner, J. D., Southwick, S. M., Johnson, D. R., Yehuda, R., & Charney, D. S. (1993). Childhood physical abuse and combat-related posttraumatic stress disorder in Vietnam veterans. *American Journal of Psychiatry, 150*, 235–239.

Bryant, R. A., Moulds, M. L., Mastrodomenico, J., Hopwood, S., Felmingham, K., & Nixon, R. D. V. (2007). Who drops out of treatment for post-traumatic stress disorder? *Clinical Psychologist, 11*, 13–15.

Burgess, A. W., & Holstrom, L. L. (1979). Rape: Sexual disruption and recovery. *American Journal of Orthopsychiatry, 49*, 648–657.

*Butterfield, M. I., McIntyre, L. M., Stechuchak, K. M., Nanda, K., & Bastian, L. A. (1998). Mental disorder symptoms in veteran women: Impact of physical and sexual assault. *Journal of the American Medical Women's Association, 53*, 198–200.

*Campbell, R., Lichty, L. F., Sturza, M., & Raja, S. (2006). Gynecological health impact of sexual assault. *Research in Nursing & Health, 29*, 399–413.

Campbell, R., & Raja, S. (1999). Secondary victimization of rape victims: Insights from mental health professionals who treat survivors of violence. *Violence and Victims, 14*, 261–275.

*Campbell, R., & Raja, S. (2005). The sexual assault and secondary victimization of female veterans: Help-seeking experiences with military and civilian social systems. *Psychology of Women Quarterly, 29*, 97–106.

*Carney, C. P., Sampson, T. R., Voelker, M., Woolson, R., Thorne, P., & Doebbeling, B. N. (2003). Women in the Gulf War: Combat experience, exposures, and subsequent health care use. *Military Medicine, 168*, 654–661.

Cason, D., Grubaugh, A. L., & Resick, P. A. (2002). Gender and PTSD treatment: Efficacy and effectiveness. In R. Kimberling, P. Ouimette, & J. Wolfe (Eds.), *Gender and PTSD* (pp. 305–334). New York, NY: Guilford Press.

*Castillo, D. T., C'De Baca, J., Conforti, K., Qualls, C., & Fallon, S. K. (2002). Anger in PTSD: General psychiatric and gender differences on the BDHI. *Journal of Loss and Trauma, 7*, 119–128.

*Chang, B., Skinner, K. M., & Boehmer, U. (2001). Religion and mental health among women veterans with sexual assault experience. *Psychiatry in Medicine, 31*, 77–95.

Chu, J. A., & Dill, D. L. (1990). Dissociative symptoms in relations to childhood physical and sexual abuse. *American Journal of Psychiatry, 14*, 887–892.

*Coyle, B. S., Wolan, D. L., & Van Horn, A. S. (1996). The prevalence of physical and sexual abuse in women veterans seeking care of a Veterans Affairs medical center. *Military Medicine, 161*, 588–593.

*Culbertson, A. L., & Rosenfeld, P. (2002). Assessment of sexual harassment in the active-duty navy. *Military Psychology, 6*, 69–93.

*David, W. S., Cotton, A. J., Simpson, T. L., & Weitlauf, J. C. (2004). Making a case for personal safety: Perceptions of vulnerability and desire for self-defense training among female veterans. *Journal of Interpersonal Violence, 19*, 991–1001.

*David, W. S., Simpson, T. L., & Cotton, A. J. (2006). Taking charge: A pilot curriculum of self-defense and personal safety training for female veterans with PTSD because of military sexual trauma. *Journal of Interpersonal Violence, 21*, 555–556.

Department of Defense. (2009). *Fiscal year 2009 annual report on sexual assault in the military*. Retrieved from http://www.sapr.mil./media/pdf/reports/fy09annualreport.pdf

DePrince, A. P. (2005). Social cognition and revictimization risk. *Journal of Trauma & Dissociation* , *6*, 125–141.

*DeRoma, V. M., Root, L., & Smith, B. S., Jr. (2003). Socioenvironmental context of sexual trauma and well-being of women veterans. *Military Medicine, 168*, 399–409.

Difede, J., Malta, L. S., Best, S., Henn-Haase, C., Metzler, T., Bryant, R., & Marmar, C. (2007). A randomized controlled clinical treatment trial for World Trade Center attack-related PTSD in disaster workers. *Journal of Nervous and Mental Disease, 195*, 861–865.

Duncan, K. (2004). *Healing from the trauma of childhood sexual abuse: The journey of women*. Connecticut: Praeger Publishers.

*Dutra, L., Grubbs, K., Greene, C., Trego, L. L., McCartin, T. L., Kloezeman, K., & Morland, L. (2011). Women at war: Implications for mental health. *Journal of Trauma & Dissociation, 12*, 25–37.

Ellis, E. M., Calhoun, K. S., & Atkeson, B. M. (1980). Sexual dysfunction in victims of rape: Victims may experience a loss of sexual arousal and frightening flashbacks even one year after assault. *Women and Health, 12*, 39–47.

*Fitzgerald, L. F., Magley, V. J., Drasgow, F., & Waldo, C. R. (1999). Measuring sexual harassment in the military: The Sexual Experiences Questionnaire (SEQ-DoD). *Military Psychology, 11*, 243–263.

Foa, E. B., Hembree, E. A., & Rothbaum, R. O. (2007). *Prolonged exposure therapy for PTSD: Emotional processing of traumatic experiences*. New York, NY: Oxford University Press.

*Fontana, A., & Rosenheck, R. (1998). Focus on women: Duty-related and sexual stress in the etiology of PTSD among women veterans who seek treatment. *Psychiatric Services, 49*, 658–662.

*Fontana, A., Schwartz, L. S., & Rosenheck, R. (1997). Posttraumatic stress disorder among female Vietnam veterans: A causal model of etiology. *American Journal of Public Health, 87*, 169–175.

Foynes, M. M., Freyd, J. J., & DePrince, A. P. (2009). Child abuse: Betrayal and disclosure. *Child Abuse and Neglect, 33*, 209–217.

*Frayne, S. M., Skinner, K. M., Sullivan, L. M., & Freund, K. M. (2003). Sexual assault while in the military: Violence as a predictor of cardiac risk? *Violence and Victims*, *18*, 219–225.

*Frayne, S. M., Skinner, K. M., Sullivan, L. M., Tripp, T. J., Hankin, C. S., Kressin, N. R., & Miller, D. R. (1999). Medical profile of women veterans administration outpatients who report a history of sexual assault occurring while in the military. *Journal of Women's Health & Gender-Based Medicine*, *8*, 835–845.

Freyd, J. J. (1996). *Betrayal trauma: The logic of forgetting childhood abuse*. Cambridge, MA: Harvard University Press.

Freyd, J. J., DePrince, A. P., & Zurbriggen, E. L. (2001). Self-reported memory for abuse depends upon victim-perpetrator relationship. *Journal of Trauma & Dissociation*, *2*, 5–17.

Freyd, J. J., Klest, B., & Allard, C. B. (2005). Betrayal trauma: Relationship to physical health, psychological distress, and a written disclosure intervention. *Journal of Trauma & Dissociation*, *6*, 83–104.

Friedman, L. S., Samet, J. H., Roberts, M. S., Hudlin, M., & Hans, P. (1992). Inquiry about victimization experiences: A survey of patient preferences and physician practices. *Archives of Internal Medicine*, 1152–1186.

*Gahm, G. A., Lucenko, B. A., Retzlaff, P., & Fukada, S. (2007). Relative impact of adverse events and screened symptoms of posttraumatic stress disorder and depression among active duty soldiers seeking mental health care. *Journal of Clinical Psychology*, *63*, 199–211.

*Goldzweig, C., Balekian, T., Rolón, C., Yano, E., & Shekelle, P. (2006). The state of women veterans' health research: Results of a systematic literature review. *Journal of General Internal Medicine*, *21*, S82–S92.

Hall, G. C. N., Hirschman, R., Graham, J. R., & Zaragoza, M. S. (1993). *Sexual aggression: Issues in etiology, assessment, and treatment*. Philadelphia, PA: Taylor & Francis.

*Hall, M. E., Sedlacek, A. R., Berenbach, J. R., & Dieckmann, N. F. (2007). Military sexual trauma services for women veterans in the Veterans Health Administration: The patient-care practice environment and perceived organizational support. *Psychological Services*, *4*, 229–238.

*Hankin, C. S., Skinner, K. M., Sullivan, L. M., Miller, D. R. Frayne, S., & Tripp, T. J. (1999). Prevalence of depressive and alcohol abuse symptoms among women VA outpatients who report experiencing sexual assault while in the military. *Journal of Traumatic Stress*, *12*, 601–612.

*Harned, M. S., & Fitzgerald, L. F. (2002). Understanding a link between sexual harassment and eating disorder symptoms: A mediational analysis. *Journal of Consulting and Clinical Psychology*, *70*, 1170–1181.

*Harned, M. S., Ormerod, A. J., Palmieri, P. A., Collinsworth, L. L. & Reed M. (2002). Sexual assault and other types of sexual harassment by workplace personnel: A comparison of antecedents and consequences. *Journal of Occupational Health Psychology*, *7*, 174–188.

*Himmelfarb, N., Yaeger, D., & Mintz, J. (2006). Posttraumatic stress disorder in female veterans with military and civilian sexual trauma. *Journal of Traumatic Stress*, *19*, 837–846.

*Houser, K. (2007). Analysis and implications of the omission of offenders in the DoD care for victims of sexual assault task force report. *Violence Against Women*, *13*, 961–970.

Jenkins, M. J., & Dambrot, F. (1987). The attribution of date rape: Observer's attitudes and sexual experiences and the dating situation. *Journal of Applied Social Psychology*, *17*, 875–895.

*Kang, H., Dalager, N., Mahan, C., & Ishii, E. (2004). The role of sexual assault on the risk of PTSD among Gulf War veterans. *Annals of Epidemiology*, *15*, 191–195.

*Katz, L. S., Bloor, L. E., Cojucar, G., & Draper, T. (2007). Women who served in Iraq seeking mental health services: Relationships between military sexual trauma, symptoms, and readjustment. *Psychological Services*, *4*, 239–249.

*Katz, L. S., Snetter, M. R., Robinson, A. H., Hewitt, P., & Cojucar, G. (2008). Holographic reprocessing: Empirical evidence to reduce posttraumatic cognitions in women veterans with PTSD from sexual trauma and abuse. *Psychotherapy Theory, Research, Practice, Training*, *45*, 186–198.

*Kelley, M. L., Schwerin, M. J., Farrar, K. L., & Lane, M. E. (2005). An evaluation of a sexual assault prevention and advocacy program for U.S. navy personnel. *Military Medicine*, *170*, 320–326.

Kessler, R. C., Sonnega, A., Bromet, E., Hughes, M., & Nelson, C. B. (1995). Posttraumatic stress disorder in the National Comorbidity Survey. *Archives in General Psychiatry*, *52*, 1048–1060.

Kilpatrick, D. (1992). *Rape in America: A report to the nation*. Charleston, SC: Crime Victims Research Center.

*Kimerling, R., Gima, K., Smith, M. W., Street, A., & Frayne, S. (2007). The Veterans Health Administration and military sexual trauma. *American Journal of Public Health*, *97*, 2160–2166.

King, D. W., King, L. A., & Foy, D. W. (1996). Prewar factors in combat-related posttraumatic stress disorder: Structural equation modeling with a national sample of female and male Vietnam veterans. *Journal of Consulting and Clinical Psychology*, *64*, 520–531.

King, D. W., King, L. A., Foy, D. W., Keane, T. M., & Fairbank, J. A. (1999). Posttraumatic stress disorder in a national sample of female and male Vietnam veterans: Risk factors, war-zone stressors, and resilience-recovery variables. *Journal of Abnormal Psychology*, *108*, 164–170.

*Leskela, J., Diepernik, M., & Kok, C. J. (2001). Group treatment with sexually assaulted male veterans: A year in review. *Group*, *25*, 303–319.

Mackey, T., Hacker, S., Weissfeld, L., Ambrose, N., Fisher, M., & Zobel, D. (1991). Comparative effects of sexual assault on sexual functioning of child sexual abuse survivors and others. *Issues in Mental Health Nursing*, *12*, 89–112.

*Magley, V. J., & Shupe, E. I. (2005). Self-labeling sexual harassment. *Sex Roles*, *53*, 173–189.

*Magley, V., Waldo, C., Drasgow, F., & Fitzgerald, L. (1999). The impact of sexual harassment on military personnel: Is it the same for men and women? *Military Psychology*, *11*(3), 283–302.

Marks, I., Lovell, K., Noshirvani, H., Livanou, M., & Thrasher, S (1998). Treatment of posttraumatic stress disorder by exposure and/or cognitive restructuring: A controlled study. *Archives of General Psychiatry*, *55*, 317–325.

*Martin, L., Rosen, L. N., Durand, D. B., Knudson, K. H., & Stretch, R. H. (2000). Psychological and physical health effects sexual assaults and nonsexual traumas among male and female United States army soldiers. *Journal of Behavioral Medicine*, *26*, 23–33.

*Martin, L., Stretch, R. H., Rosen, L. N., Knudson, K. H., & Durand, D. B. (1998). Prevalence and timing of sexual assaults in a sample of male and female U.S. army soldiers. *Military Medicine*, *163*, 213–216.

Matthieu, M., & Ivanoff, A. (2006). Treatment of human-caused trauma: Attrition in the adult outcomes research. *Journal of Interpersonal Violence*, *21*, 1654–1664.

*McCall-Hosenfeld, J. S., Liebschutz, J. M., Spiro, A., & Seaver, M. R. (2009). Sexual assault in the military and its impact on sexual satisfaction in women veterans: A proposed model. *Journal of Women's Health*, *18*, 901–909.

Merrill, L. L., Newell, C. E., Milner, J. S., Koss, M. P., Hervig, L. L., Gold, S. R., . . . Thornton, S. R. (1998). Prevalence of pre-military adult sexual victimization and aggression in a navy recruit sample. *Military Medicine*, *163* 209–212.

Merrill, L. L., Thomsen, C. J., Gold, S. R., & Milner, J. S. (2001). Childhood abuse and premilitary sexual assault in male navy recruits. *Journal of Consulting and Clinical Psychology*, *69*, 252–261.

*Monson, C. M., Schnurr, P., Resick, P. A., Friedman, M. J., Young-Xu, Y., & Stevens, S. P. (2006). Cognitive processing therapy for veterans with military-related posttraumatic stress disorder. *Journal of Consulting and Clinical Psychology*, *74*, 898–907.

*Murdoch, M., Hodges, J., Hunt, C., Cowper, D., Kressin, N., & O'Brien, N. (2003). Gender differences in service connection for PTSD. *Medical Care*, *41*, 950–961.

*Murdoch, M., & Nichol, K. L. (1995). Women veteran's experiences with domestic violence and sexual harassment while in the military. *Archives of Family Medicine*, *4*, 411–418.

*Murdoch, M., Polusny, M. A., Hodges, J., & Cowper, D. (2006). The association between in-service sexual harassment and posttraumatic stress disorder among Department of Veterans Affairs disability applicants. *Military Medicine*, *171*, 166–173.

*Murdoch, M., Polusny, M. A., Hodges, J., & O'Brien, N. (2004). Prevalence of in-service and post-service sexual assault among combat and noncombat veterans applying for Department of Veterans Affairs posttraumatic stress disorder disability benefits. *Military Medicine*, *169*, 392–395.

*Murdoch, M., Pryor, J. B., Polusny, M. A., & Gackstetter, G. D. (2007). Function and psychiatric symptoms among military men and women exposed to sexual stressors. *Military Medicine*, *172*, 718–725.

Mynatt, C. R., & Allgeier, E. R. (1990). Risk factors, self attributions and adjustment problems among victims of sexual coercion. *Journal of Applied Social Psychology*, *20*, 130–153.

*Newell, C. E., Rosenfeld, P., & Cullertson, A. L. (1995). Sexual harassment experiences and equal opportunity perception of navy women. *Sex Roles*, *32*, 159–168.

Norris, F. H. (1992). Epidemiology of trauma: Frequency and impact of different potentially traumatic events on different demographic groups. *Journal of Consulting and Clinical Psychology*, *60*, 409–418.

*O'Brien, C., Gaher, R. M., Pope, C., & Smiley, P. (2008). Difficulty identifying feelings predicts the persistence of trauma symptoms in a sample of veterans who experienced military sexual trauma. *Journal of Nervous and Mental Disease*, *196*, 252–255.

Persons, J. B., Burns, D. D., & Perloff, J. M. (1988). Predictors of dropout and outcome in cognitive therapy for depression in a private practice setting. *Cognitive Therapy & Research*, *12*, 557–575.

Plattner, B., Silvermann, M. A., Redlich, A. D., Carrion, V. G., Feucht, M., Friedrich, M. H., & Steiner, H. (2003). Pathways to dissociation: Intrafamilial versus extrafamilial trauma in juvenile delinquents. *Journal of Nervous and Mental Disease*, *191*, 781–788.

*Raiha, N. K. (1983). Comprehensive care for the victim of sexual assault. *Military Medicine*, *148*, 796–799.

*Rauch, S. A. M., Defever, E., Favorite, T., Duro, A., Garrity, C., Martis, B., & Liberzon, I. (2009). Prolonged exposure for PTSD in a Veterans Health Administration PTSD clinic. *Journal of Traumatic Stress*, *22*, 60–64.

Resick, P. A., & Schnicke, M. K. (1992). Cognitive processing therapy for sexual assault victims. *Journal of Consulting and Clinical Psychology*, *60*, 748–756.

*Ritchie, E. C. (1998). Reactions to rape: A military forensic psychiatrist's perspective. *Military Medicine*, *163*, 505–508.

*Rosen, L. N., & Martin, L. (1998a). Childhood maltreatment history as a risk factor for sexual harassment among U.S. army soldiers. *Violence and Victims*, *13*, 269–286.

*Rosen, L. N., & Martin, L. (1998b). Predictors of tolerance of sexual harassment among male U.S. army soldiers. *Violence Against Women*, *4*, 491–504.

Roth, S., Newman, E., Pelcovitz, D., van der Kolk, B., & Mandel, F. S. (1997). Complex PTSD in victims exposed to sexual and physical abuse: Results from the *DSM-IV* field trial for posttraumatic stress disorder. *Journal of Traumatic Stress*, *10*, 539–556.

*Sadler, A. G., Booth, B. M., Cook, B. L., & Doebbeling, B. N. (2003). Factors associated with women's risk of rape in the military environment. *American Journal of Industrial Medicine*, *43*, 262–273.

*Sadler, A. G., Booth, B. M., Cook, B. L., Torner, J. C., & Doebbeling, B. N. (2001). The military environment: Risk factors for women's non-fatal assaults. *Journal of Occupational and Environmental Medicine*, *43*, 325–334.

*Sadler, A. G., Booth, B. M., Mengeling, M. A., & Doebbeling, B. N. (2004). Life span and repeated violence against women during military service: Effects on health status and outpatient utilization. *Journal of Women's Health*, *13*, 799–811.

*Sadler, A. G., Booth, B. M., Nielson, D., & Doebbeling, B. N. (2000). Health-related consequences of physical and sexual violence: Women in the military. *Obstetrics and Gynecology*, *96*, 473–480.

*Schnurr, P. P., Friedman, M. J., Engel., C. C., Foa, E. B., Shea, M. T., Chow, B. K., . . . Bernardy, N. (2007). Cognitive behavioral therapy for posttraumatic stress disorder in women: A randomized controlled trial. *Journal of the American Medical Association*, *297*, 820–830.

Schottenbauer, M. A., Glass, C. R., Arnkoff, D. B., Tendick, V., & Gray, S. H. (2008). Nonresponse and dropout rates in outcome studies on PTSD: Review and methodological considerations. *Psychiatry: Interpersonal and Biological Process*, *71*, 134–168.

Schultz, J. R., Kathryn, M. B., Naugle, A. E., & Polusny, M. A. (2006). Child sexual abuse and adulthood sexual assault among military veteran and civilian women. *Military Medicine*, *171*, 723–728.

Shannon, L., Logan, T. K., Cole, J., & Walker, R. (2008). An examination of women's alcohol use and partner victimization experiences among women with protective orders. *Substance Use and Misuse*, *43*, 1110–1128.

Sharf, J. (2008). Psychotherapy dropout: A meta-analytic review of premature termination. *Dissertation Abstracts International: Section B: The Sciences and Engineering*, *68*, 6336.

*Shipherd, J. C., Pineles, S. L., Gradus, J. L., & Resick, P. A. (2009). Sexual harassment in the marines, posttraumatic stress symptoms, and perceived health: Evidence for sex differences. *Journal of Traumatic Stress*, *22*, 3–10.

Siegel, J. M., Golding, J. M., Stein, J. A., Burnam, M. A., & Sorenson, S. B. (1990). Reactions to sexual assault: A community study. *Journal of Interpersonal Violence*, *5*, 229–246.

*Skinner, K. M., Kressin, N., Frayne, S., Tripp, T. J., Hankin, C. S., Miller, D. R., & Sullivan, L. M. (2000). The prevalence of military sexual assault among female Veterans' Administration outpatients. *Journal of Interpersonal Violence*, *15*, 291–310.

*Smith, D. W., Frueh, C. F., Sawchuk, C. N., & Johnson, M. R. (1999). Relationship between symptom over-reporting and pre- and post-combat trauma history in veterans evaluated for PTSD. *Depression & Anxiety*, *10*, 119–124.

*Stark, S., Chernyshenko, O. S., Lancaster, A. R., Drasgow, F., & Fitzgerald, L. F. (2002). Toward standardized measurement of sexual harassment: Shortening the SEQ-DoD using item response theory. *Military Psychology*, *14*, 49–72.

Steel, Z., Jones, J., Adcock, S., Clancy, R., Bridgeford-West, L., & Austin, J. (2000). Why the high rate of dropout from individualized cognitive–behavior therapy for bulimia nervosa? *International Journal of Eating Disorders*, *28*, 209–214.

Stein, M. B., Lang, A. J., Laffaye, C., Satz, L. E., Lenox, R. J., & Dresselhaus, T. R. (2004). Relationship of sexual assault history to somatic symptoms and health anxiety in women. *General Hospital of Psychiatry*, *26*, 178–183.

Steury, S., Spencer, S., & Parkinson, G. W. (2004). The social context of recovery. *Psychiatry: Interpersonal and Biological Processes*, *67*, 158–163.

*Street, A. E., Gradus, J. L., Stafford, J., & Kelly, K. (2007). Gender differences in experiences of sexual harassment: Data from a male-dominated environment. *Journal of Consulting and Clinical Psychology*, *75*, 464–474.

*Street, A. E., Stafford, J., Mahan, C. M., & Hendricks, A. (2008). Sexual harassment and assault experienced by reservists during military service: Prevalence and health correlates. *Journal of Rehabilitation Research & Development*, *45*, 409–420.

Suliman, S., Mkabile, S. G., Fincham, D. S., Ahmed, R., Stein, D. J., & Seedat, S. (2009). Cumulative effect of multiple traumas on symptoms of posttraumatic stress disorder, anxiety and depression in adolescents. *Comprehensive Psychiatry*, *50*, 121–127.

*Suris, A. M., Davis, L. L., Kashner, T. M., Gillaspy, J. A., Jr., & Petty, F. (1998). A survey of sexual trauma treatment provided by VA medical centers. *Psychiatric Services*, *49*, 382–384.

*Suris, A., & Lind, L. (2008). Military sexual trauma: A review of prevalence and associated health consequences in veterans. *Trauma, Violence, & Abuse*, *9*, 250–269.

*Suris, A., Lind, L., Kashner, T. M., & Borman, P. D. (2007). Mental health, quality of life and health functioning in women veterans: Differential outcomes associated with military and civilian sexual assault. *Journal of Interpersonal Violence*, *22*, 179–197.

*Suris, A., Lind, L., Kashner, T. M., Borman, P. D., & Petty, F. (2004). Sexual assault in women veterans: An examination of PTSD risk, health care utilization and cost of care. *Psychosomatic Medicine*, *66*, 749–756.

Tarrier, N., & Humphreys, A. L. (2003). PTSD and the social support of the interpersonal environment: The development of social cognitive behavior therapy. *Journal of Cognitive Psychotherapy*, *17*, 187–198.

Testa, M., VanZile-Tamsen, C., & Livingston, J. (2007). Prospective prediction of women's sexual victimization by intimate and nonintimate male perpetrators. *Journal of Consulting and Clinical Psychology*, *75*, 52–60.

Tjaden, P., & Thoennes, N. (2000). *Full report of the prevalence, incidence, and consequences of violence against women: Findings from the National Violence Against Women Survey* (Publication No. NCJ 183781). Washington, DC: National Institute of Justice and the Centers for Disease Control and Prevention. Retrieved from http://www.ncjrs.gov/pdffiles1/nig/183781.pdf

U.S. Merit Systems Protection Board. (1995). *Sexual harassment in the federal government: Trends, progress, continuing challenges*. Washington DC: U.S. Government Printing Office.

*Valente, S., & Wright, C. (2007). Military sexual trauma: Violence and sexual abuse. *Military Medicine*, *172*, 259–265.

van der Kolk, B. A., Roth, S., Pelcovitz, D., Sunday, S., & Spinazzola, J. (2005). Disorders of extreme stress: The empirical foundation of a complex adaptation to trauma. *Journal of Traumatic Stress*, *18*, 389–399.

Veteran's Benefits: Counseling and Treatment for Sexual Trauma, 38 U.S.C. § 1720D (1992).

*Vickerman, K. A., & Margolin, G. (2009). Rape treatment outcome research: Empirical findings and state of literature. *Clinical Psychological Review*, *29*, 431–448.

*Vogt, D., Bruce, T. A., Street, A. E., & Stafford, J. (2007). Attitudes toward women and tolerance for sexual harassment among reservists. *Violence Against Women*, *13*, 879–900.

*Vogt, D. S., Pless, A. P., King, L. A., & King, D. W. (2005). Erratum for deployment stressors, gender, and mental health outcomes among Gulf War I veterans. *Journal of Traumatic Stress*, *18*, 115–127.

*Waldfogel, S., & Mueser, K. T. (1988). Another case of chronic PTSD with auditory hallucinations. *American Journal of Psychiatry*, *145*, 1314.

Waller, G. (1997). Drop-out and failure to engage in individual outpatient cognitive behavior therapy for bulimic disorders. *International Journal of Eating Disorders*, *22*, 35–41.

Widom, C. S., & Morris, S. M. (1997). Accuracy of adult recollections of childhood victimization, part 2: Childhood sexual abuse. *Psychological Assessment*, *9*, 34–53.

Williams, L. M. (1994). Recall of childhood trauma: A prospective study of women's memories of child sexual abuse. *Journal of Consult Clinical Psychology*, *62*, 1167–1176.

*Wolfe, J., Sharkansky, E. J., Read, J. P., Dawson, R., Martin, J. A., & Ouimette, P. C. (1998). Sexual harassment and assault as predictors of PTSD symptomatology among U.S. female Persian Gulf war military personnel. *Journal of Interpersonal Violence*, *13*, 40–57.

*Yaeger, D., Himmelfarb, N., Cammack, A., & Mintz, J. (2006). *DSM-IV* diagnosed posttraumatic stress disorder in women veterans with and without military sexual trauma. *Journal of General Internal Medicine*, *21*, S65–S69.

*Young, S. A. (1995). Rape trauma syndrome in the military courts. *Bulletin of the American Academy of Psychiatry and the Law*, *23*, 563–671

Zayfert, C., DeVivia, J. C., Becker, C. B., Pike, J. L., Gillock, K. L., & Hayes, S. A. (2005). Exposure utilization and completion of cognitive behavioral therapy for PTSD in a real world clinical practice. *Journal of Traumatic Stress*, *18*, 637–645.

*Zinzow, H. M., Grubaugh, A. L., Monnier, J., Suffoletta-Maierle, S., & Frueh, B. C. (2007). Trauma among female veterans: A critical review. *Trauma, Violence, & Abuse*, *8*, 384–400.

Index

Page numbers in *Italics* represent tables.
Page numbers followed by a represent appendix.